Concise Guide to Pediatric Arrhythmias

Concise Guide to Pediatric Arrhythmias

Christopher Wren, PhD

Consultant Pediatric Cardiologist
Freeman Hospital (NHS)
Newcastle upon Tyne
UK

WILEY-BLACKWELL

A John Wiley & Sons, Ltd., Publication

This edition first published 2012 © 2012 by John Wiley & Sons Ltd.

Wiley-Blackwell is an imprint of John Wiley & Sons, formed by the merger of Wiley's global Scientific, Technical and Medical business with Blackwell Publishing.

Registered office: John Wiley & Sons, Ltd, The Atrium, Southern Gate, Chichester, West Sussex, PO19 8SQ, UK

Editorial offices: 9600 Garsington Road, Oxford, OX4 2DQ, UK

The Atrium, Southern Gate, Chichester, West Sussex, PO19 8SQ, UK

111 River Street, Hoboken, NJ 07030-5774, USA

For details of our global editorial offices, for customer services and for information about how to apply for permission to reuse the copyright material in this book please see our website at www.wiley.com/wiley-blackwell

Library of Congress Cataloging-in-Publication Data
Wren, C. (Christopher)
   Concise guide to pediatric arrhythmias / Christopher Wren.
      p. ; cm.
   Includes bibliographical references and index.
   ISBN-13: 978-0-470-65855-0 (pbk. : alk. paper)
   ISBN-10: 0-470-65855-X (pbk. : alk. paper)
1. Arrhythmia in children–Handbooks, manuals, etc.   I. Title.
   [DNLM: 1. Arrhythmias, Cardiac–diagnosis–Handbooks.   2. Arrhythmias,
Cardiac–therapy–Handbooks.   3. Child.   4. Infant. WS 39]
   RJ426.A7W74 2012
   618.92′128–dc23

                                                        2011015325

A catalogue record for this book is available from the British Library.

This book is published in the following electronic formats: ePDF 9781119979456; Wiley Online Library 9781119979487; ePub 9781119979463; Mobi 9781119979470

Set in 9/12pt Meridien by Aptara® Inc., New Delhi, India

1   2012

Contents

Foreword

I was particularly honored when Dr. Wren asked me to write this brief foreword to his monograph, *"A Concise Guide to Pediatric Arrhythmias"*. However, when I reflected on this opportunity, I wondered whether there was a deeper motivation to Dr. Wren's request. Not noted for my prowess in electrophysiology, I wonder whether he felt it long overdue that I be educated in the causes, identification and treatment of electrical disturbances of the heart!

While primarily aimed at the non-specialist, and trainee, Dr. Wren's book will provide an important resource to anyone caring for children with heart disease. Anyone that knows Dr. Wren will attest to his simple, pragmatic, and insightful approach to problems, his huge wealth of clinical experience, and his scholarly and critical approach to his own written works, and those of others. This book is a perfect reflection of those attributes, providing the reader with a beautifully written, easily assimilated, and clinically oriented approach to electrophysiology. While every illustration has an important message, and every paragraph is rich in content, the message never becomes overwhelming. Complex basic concepts are handled with a light touch, and the reader is guided through potentially complicated diagnostic and management algorithms with a logical, sequential, and thoughtfully outlined rationale. As such, it is the perfect text for those in training, a go-to resource for the generalist, or handy aide memoire to those of us who are more senior.

So, whether intended or not, I have indeed been educated by reading Dr. Wren's *"Concise Guide to Pediatric Arrhythmias"*. I am certain that those likewise exposed to this book will be similarly enlightened. Indeed, I am sure it will rapidly become required reading and a staple text in our field.

Andrew Redington
Head of Cardiology
The Hospital for Sick Children
Toronto, ON
Canada

Preface

Most infants and children with arrhythmias present to a pediatrician before being referred to a pediatric cardiologist for assessment and management. Thus, the pediatrician has to be able to recognize the arrhythmia and in some cases to provide the acute treatment. Other arrhythmias arise in children who are already under the care of a cardiologist – either as part of the natural history of their heart problem or as a consequence of its treatment. This book is intended to be useful to pediatric trainees and pediatricians with an interest in cardiology as well as to trainees in and practitioners of pediatric cardiology and pediatric intensive care. It aims to provide a guide to the recognition of arrhythmias and their management. It is not written for the specialist because there are already plenty of advanced works written by experts for experts. It contains no invasive electrophysiological images but does give a brief guide to how and when invasive study might be indicated as well as an introductory guide to the use of catheter ablation and pacemakers and defibrillators.

I am indebted to many colleagues who have referred patients or who have helped to source some of the ECG examples. They include John O'Sullivan, Richard Kirk, and Milind Chaudhari in Freeman Hospital, Newcastle upon Tyne and Philip Rees and Martin Lowe in Great Ormond Street Hospital, London. I am also grateful to Andrew Sands, Satish Adwani, Kevin Walsh, Paul Oslizlok, Desmond Duff, Frank Casey, and Karen McLeod, and I am sure there are others, who have given permission to use images from patients who they have referred.

The quality of the ECGs that we have available for analysis varies and is sometimes less than ideal. However, if the only traces we have are from a paramedic recording or from a Holter recording or arrive via fax, they may still provide valuable information. I have chosen the best examples I have of all the various arrhythmias but they are all real ECGs so their quality also varies. They do represent the situations that we are faced with in real life and are preferable to redrawn idealized images.

The layout of the book is perhaps a little different from a traditional textbook with a great emphasis on ECG examples. Many of the individual arrhythmias are discussed in a small number of pages so that all the key features are available almost at a glance.

I have tried to limit the number of abbreviations in the text because they may be confusing for readers whose first language is not English. However, some are inevitable and most will be fairly familiar, such as AV, BBB, and WPW. A list of abbreviations is provided.

The opinions on antiarrhythmic drug treatment discussed throughout the book are my own and represent a fairly Eurocentric view. I recognize that practice varies in other parts of the world and other approaches to drug treatment are adopted. It is not possible to present all options for treatment but it is probably true to say that almost all antiarrhythmic drugs have been used for the treatment of almost all arrhythmias at some stage.

Over the past few years I have given many lectures, talks, seminars, and courses on the subjects of ECG interpretation and cardiac arrhythmias in infants and children, and in young adults with congenital heart disease. I have been consistently impressed by the interest and enthusiasm of those whom I have met, many of whom have asked for a monograph such as this. I hope that this will meet the need.

Christopher Wren
2011

Abbreviations

AAVRT	antidromic atrioventricular re-entry tachycardia	**FAT**	focal atrial tachycardia
AET	atrial ectopic tachycardia	**HBT**	His bundle tachycardia
AF	atrial fibrillation	**JET**	junctional ectopic tachycardia
AFL	atrial flutter	**LBBB**	left bundle branch block
AFRT	atriofascicular re-entry tachycardia	**LQTS**	long QT syndrome
AT	atrial tachycardia	**MAT**	multifocal atrial tachycardia
AV	atrioventricular	**OAVRT**	orthodromic atrioventricular re-entry tachycardia
AVB	atrioventricular block	**PJRT**	permanent junctional reciprocating tachycardia
AVNRT	atrioventricular nodal re-entry tachycardia		
AVRT	atrioventricular re-entry tachycardia	**RBBB**	right bundle branch block
BBB	bundle branch block	**SR**	sinus rhythm
CAT	chaotic atrial tachycardia	**ST**	sinus tachycardia
CAVB	complete atrioventricular block	**SVT**	supraventricular tachycardia
CPVT	catecholaminergic polymorphic ventricular tachycardia	**VT**	ventricular tachycardia
		WPW	Wolff–Parkinson–White

1 Anatomy, physiology, and epidemiology of arrhythmias

An arrhythmia is an abnormality of cardiac rhythm. Arrhythmias differ in their population frequency, anatomical substrate, physiological mechanism, etiology, natural history, prognostic significance, and response to treatment. As is emphasized throughout this book, it is important to gain as much information as possible about the substrate and mechanism of an arrhythmia to be able to predict the natural history and to define the prognosis and response to treatment.

Electrical anatomy of the normal heart

The diagram in Figure 1.1 shows a sketch of the electrically active parts of the normal heart. The atrial muscle and ventricular muscle are separated by insulation of the fibrous mitral and tricuspid valve rings, and normally the only connection between them is via the His bundle.

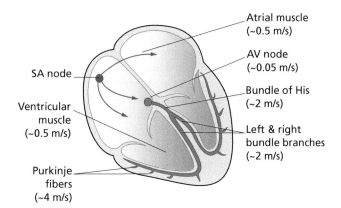

Figure 1.1

All cardiac myocytes are capable of electrical conduction and have intrinsic pacemaker activity. Each tissue has a conduction velocity and a refractory period, both of which vary with changes in heart rate and influences such as autonomic tone, circulating catecholamines, etc. The conduction velocities of various parts of the heart vary as shown in Figure 1.1.

Basic mechanisms of tachycardias

Although it is not necessary to have a deep understanding of cardiac electrophysiology to diagnose and treat a cardiac arrhythmia, some knowledge of the basics is helpful. Tachycardias are mostly caused by re-entry or abnormal automaticity. Some

Concise Guide to Pediatric Arrhythmias, First Edition. Christopher Wren.
© 2012 John Wiley & Sons, Ltd. Published 2012 by John Wiley & Sons, Ltd.

common examples are shown in Figure 1.2. A few rare types of tachycardia are probably caused by a third mechanism, triggered activity.

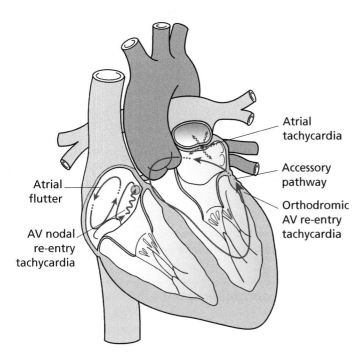

Atrial
tachycardia

Accessory
pathway

Orthodromic
AV re-entry
tachycardia

Atrial
flutter

AV nodal
re-entry
tachycardia

Figure 1.2

Many common tachycardias are caused by *re-entry*. This means that there is a self-propagating wave of electrical excitation which maintains the arrhythmia. The fundamental requirements for re-entry are that there should be: (1) an anatomical circuit, (2) a zone of slow conduction in the circuit, and (3) a region of unidirectional block. The best model of re-entry is an orthodromic atrioventricular (AV) re-entry, e.g. Wolff–Parkinson–White syndrome (see Chapter 13). The circuit comprises the accessory pathway, atrium, AV node, and ventricle. The slow conduction is in the AV node and functional unidirectional block can occur in the accessory pathway. Tachycardia is interrupted if one part of the circuit has a refractory period longer than the cycle length of the tachycardia. In practice this is most easily achieved by prolonging AV node refractoriness with adenosine. Tachycardia will restart only if the requirements for reinitiation are met. These include a trigger (often an atrial or ventricular premature beat) and an appropriate balance of electrical behavior of the various parts of the circuit. Re-entry tachycardias can be started and stopped by pacing and stopped by cardioversion. Other examples of re-entry include AV nodal re-entry tachycardia (see Chapter 16), atrial flutter (see Chapter 9), and some types of ventricular tachycardia (see Chapter 18).

Fewer tachycardias are caused by *abnormal automaticity*. The best model of automaticity is sinus rhythm. Similar to sinus rhythm, automatic (also known as ectopic) tachycardias cannot be started or stopped by pacing and cannot be interrupted by cardioversion. In the normal heart the sinus node has the highest spontaneous rate and, therefore, determines the rhythm. If the sinus node fails another part of the heart with a lower pacemaker rate, usually the AV node, will provide an escape rhythm. Sometimes an area of the heart other than the sinus node will have an abnormally high spontaneous rate and will produce an automatic (or ectopic) tachycardia, overriding the sinus node. Examples of tachycardias caused by enhanced automaticity include atrial ectopic tachycardia (a type of focal atrial tachycardia – see Chapter 7), junctional ectopic tachycardia (see Chapter 17), and some types of ventricular tachycardia (see Chapter 18).

Triggered activity is the least common tachycardia mechanism. Depolarization is caused by a trigger – either an early after-depolarization or a delayed after-depolarization. Triggered activity causes ventricular arrhythmias in long QT syndrome, some electrolyte disturbances, and in some postoperative ventricular tachycardia with myocardial injury.

Basic mechanisms of bradycardias

Bradycardias are due to either failure of impulse generation or failure of conduction. The most common example of failure of impulse generation is sinoatrial disease (see Chapter 30). Abnormal sinus node function may be due extrinsic effects (high vagal tone) or to depressed automaticity. Significant bradycardias are more commonly due to second- or third-degree AV block (see Chapters 28 and 29).

Epidemiology of arrhythmias

Some arrhythmias are more common than others but there are almost no data on the population prevalence of these conditions. However, we recognize that the prevalence and spectrum of arrhythmias change with age. Faced with a new patient with an arrhythmia, our diagnosis is based mainly on the child's age, the age of onset of arrhythmia, the history (palpitations, heart failure, syncope, etc.), and the ECG findings. but should also take into account the prevalence of different arrhythmias (in other words, a common arrhythmia is often a more likely diagnosis than a rare one).

Probably fewer than half of new tachycardias present in the first year of life. By far the most common tachycardia presenting in early infancy is orthodromic AV re-entry (see Chapter 12). Most of these infants have a normal ECG in sinus rhythm but some show ventricular pre-excitation. Other neonatal tachycardias are much less common and include atrial flutter (see Chapter 9), permanent junctional reciprocating tachycardia (see Chapter 14), atrial tachycardia (see Chapter 7), and ventricular tachycardia (see Chapters 19 and 20).

The most common tachycardia in childhood is also orthodromic AV re-entry tachycardia, although AV nodal re-entry tachycardia (see Chapter 16) becomes progressively more common after the age of 5 years. Less common tachycardias in this age group are antidromic AV re-entry (see Chapter 13), atriofascicular re-entry (see Chapter 15), ventricular tachycardias (see Chapter 18), and atrial tachycardias (see Chapter 7).

Arrhythmias presenting with palpitations include most of the common types of supraventricular tachycardia and a few cases of ventricular tachycardia. Many children with palpitations do not have an arrhythmia and a detailed first-hand history is essential before assessing the likelihood of an arrhythmia and the necessity of further investigation. Similarly very few children with chest pain have arrhythmias (or indeed any cardiac abnormality) and only a few with syncope have an arrhythmia. Again it all depends on the history.

Incessant tachycardias presenting with heart failure or apparent cardiomyopathy include focal atrial tachycardia (see Chapter 7), permanent junctional reciprocating tachycardia (see Chapter 14), incessant idiopathic infant ventricular tachycardia (see Chapter 20), and orthodromic atrioventricular re-entry tachycardia (see Chapter 15).

Arrhythmias presenting with syncope include complete AV block (see Chapter 29), atrial fibrillation in Wolff–Parkinson–White syndrome (see Chapter 13), sinoatrial disease (see Chapter 30), and ventricular tachycardia, especially in long QT syndrome (see Chapter 25), catecholaminergic ventricular tachycardia (see Chapter 26) or late after cardiac surgery (see Chapter 32). Syncope is discussed in detail in Chapter 35.

Some arrhythmias are so common as to be considered as almost normal variants. They include atrial premature beats (see Chapter 11), ventricular premature beats (see Chapter 23), and transient nocturnal Wenckebach AV block (see Chapter 28).

Arrhythmias occurring early or late after cardiac surgery are specific to those situations and are considered in detail in Chapters 31 and 32, respectively.

Key references

Anderson RH, Ho SY. The morphologic substrates for pediatric arrhythmias. *Cardiol Young* 1991; **1**:159–76.

Antzelevitch C. Basic mechanisms of reentrant arrhythmias. *Curr Opin Cardiol* 2001;**16**:1–7.

Kantoch MJ. Supraventricular tachycardia in children. *Indian J Pediatr* 2005;**72**:609–19.

Ko JK, Deal BJ, Strasburger JF, et al. Supraventricular tachycardia mechanisms and their age distribution in pediatric patients. *Am J Cardiol* 1992;**69**:1028–32.

Massin MM, Benatar A, Rondia G. Epidemiology and outcome of tachyarrhythmias in tertiary pediatric cardiac centers. *Cardiology* 2008;**111**:191–6.

Mazgalev TN, Ho SY, Anderson RH. Anatomic-electrophysiological correlations concerning the pathways for atrio-ventricular conduction. *Circulation* 2001;**103**:2660–7.

Paul T, Bertram H, Bökenkamp R, et al. Supraventricular tachycardia in infants, children and adolescents: diagnosis, and pharmacological and interventional therapy. *Paediatr Drugs* 2000;**2**:171–81.

Porter MJ, Morton JB, Denman R, et al. Influence of age and gender on the mechanism of supraventricular tachycardia. *Heart Rhythm* 2004;**1**:393–6.

Sekar RP. Epidemiology of arrhythmias in children. *Indian Pacing Electrophysiol J* 2008;**8** (suppl 1):S8–3.

Tipple MA. Usefulness of the electrocardiogram in diagnosing mechanisms of tachycardia. *Pediatr Cardiol* 2000;**21**:516–21.

2 ECGs and other recording devices

The 12-lead ECG

The ECG is conventionally recorded at a speed of 25 mm/s and at a calibration of 1 cm = 1 mV. A standard 12-lead ECG includes three standard (bipolar) limb leads – I, II, and III – three augmented unipolar limb leads – aVR, aVL, and aVF – and six unipolar chest leads – V1–V6. Accurate positioning of the leads (especially the chest leads) is important, as shown in Figure 2.1. V1 and V2 are in the fourth intercostal space, V4 is in the fifth intercostal space in the midclavicular line, V5 is in the anterior axillary line, and V6 in the midaxillary line, both these last two horizontal to V4.

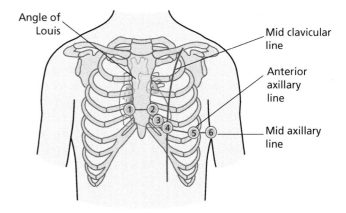

Figure 2.1

Routine evaluation of an ECG involves assessment of the heart rate, heart rhythm, and QRS axis, then the P waves, QRS complexes, T waves, and measurement of the PR, QRS, and QT intervals. Many modern ECG machines automatically measure and display many of these variables. The measurements are usually accurate and reliable but a machine-derived interpretation of the ECG should be treated with some caution, even if it is produced by a pediatric algorithm. The machine often distinguishes between normality and abnormality fairly accurately (assuming that the age of the patient is entered into the algorithm) but analysis of the type of arrhythmia is often unreliable.

The importance of a 12-lead ECG is illustrated in Figure 2.2, which shows obvious pre-excitation. However, careful analysis of the 12-lead recording shows deep negative delta waves in inferior leads, characteristic of an accessory pathway situated in the coronary sinus. Whenever possible, a 12-lead ECG recording in sinus rhythm and during symptoms should be obtained in children with suspected or proven arrhythmia.

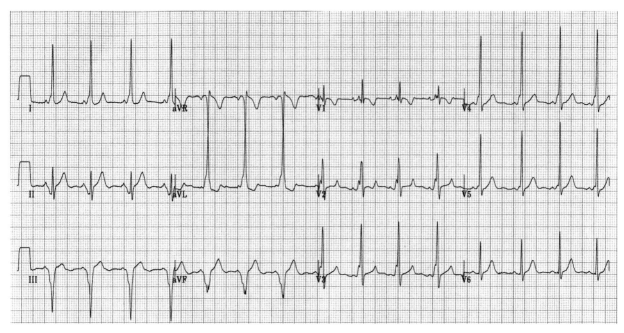

Figure 2.2

Rhythm strips

Rhythm strips are most useful in documenting changes in rhythm in response to interventions such as adenosine administration, but they should not be seen as an alternative to recording a 12-lead ECG. Rhythm strips usually contain three leads but, on some machines, there may be six, twelve, or only one. The leads selected vary. Leads I, aVF, and V1 are a good combination but others may be preferred after examining the 12-lead ECG. Figure 2.3 shows a rhythm strip of the response of atrial flutter to adenosine administration with the production of variable AV conduction (see Chapter 9).

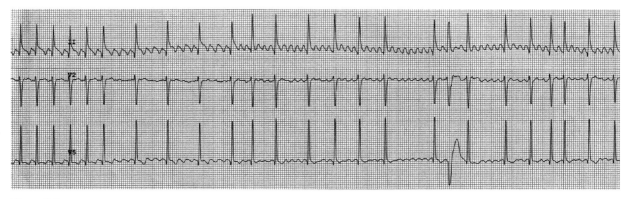

Figure 2.3

Ambulatory ECG recording

Holter monitoring, or ambulatory ECG recording, has become a standard test in the investigation and follow-up of children with suspected or proven arrhythmias. It is well tolerated and particularly useful in children with fairly frequent symptoms, suggesting that there is a reasonable chance of recording the ECG during symptoms. It is also valuable in assessing response to treatment in children with incessant tachycardias, congenital long QT syndrome, etc. The recording in Figure 2.4 comes from a young child with a history of frequent syncope. The history suggested a diagnosis of reflex asystolic syncope. The ECG shows transient atrioventricular (AV) block with ventricular standstill and a pause of 4.8 s. This event was not associated with symptoms. The extra yield from longer periods of continuous recording is low.

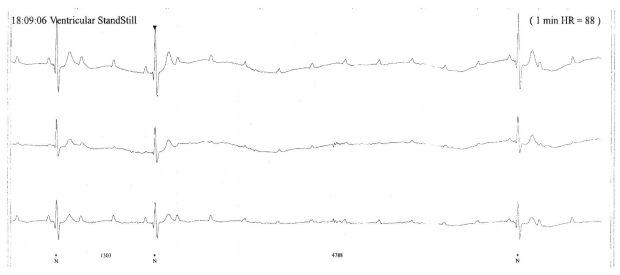

Figure 2.4

ECG event recorders

Event recorders are carried by children or their parents but are not necessarily worn all the time. They can be used in loop mode (where they are worn constantly and a button is pressed during symptoms to make a record of the ECG) or event mode (when the recorder is applied and a recording made when symptoms occur). Figure 2.5 shows a recording from a girl with recurrent syncope who was found to have catecholaminergic polymorphic ventricular tachycardia.

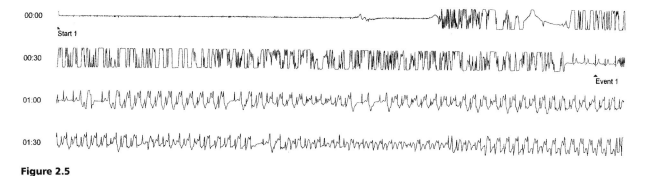

Figure 2.5

Exercise ECG

Treadmill or bicycle exercise ECG recording is sometimes helpful in investigation of arrhythmias but is useful in providing reassurance for children and their families in the presence of exercise-related symptoms thought not to be due to arrhythmia. Exercise-induced arrhythmias are unusual but are sometimes seen in AV re-entry or

AV nodal re-entry. The exercise test is very helpful in suspected catecholaminergic polymorphic ventricular tachycardia (see Chapter 26).

Key references

Davignon A, Rautaharju P, Boisselle E, et al. Normal ECG standards for infants and children. *Pediatr Cardiol* 1979–80;**1**:123–52.

Dickinson DF. The normal ECG in childhood and adolescence. *Heart* 2005;**91**:1626–30.

Garson A Jr. *The Electrocardiogram in Infants and Children: A systematic approach.* Philadelphia: Lea & Febiger, 1983.

Kadish AH, Buxton AE, Kennedy HL, et al. ACC/AHA clinical competence statement on electrocardiography and ambulatory electrocardiography. *Circulation* 2001;**104**:3169–78.

Kinlay S, Leitch JW, Neil A, et al. Cardiac event recorders yield more diagnoses and are more cost-effective than 48-hour Holter monitoring in patients with palpitations. A controlled clinical trial. *Ann Intern Med* 1996;**124**:16–20.

Paridon SM, Alpert BS, Boas SR, et al. Clinical stress testing in the pediatric age group: A statement from the American Heart Association Council on cardiovascular disease in the young, committee on atherosclerosis, hypertension, and obesity in youth. *Circulation* 2006;**113**;1905–20.

Rijnbeek PR, Witsenburg M, Schrama E, et al. New normal limits for the paediatric electrocardiogram. *Eur Heart J* 2001;**22**:702–11.

Tipple M. Interpretation of electrocardiograms in infants and children. *Images Paediatr Cardiol* 1999;**1**:3–13. Available at: www.health.gov.mt/impaedcard/issue/issue1/ipc00103.htm#top (accessed 20 May 2011).

3 Other diagnostic techniques

Implanted loop recorder

In children with worrying syncope but no proven diagnosis, an implanted loop recorder may be very helpful. The device has a 3-year battery and is inserted subcutaneously in the left axilla or on the left anterior chest wall. It works in loop mode and can be programmed to store recordings of arrhythmias which have rates below or above preset limits. A recording can also be triggered by children or their parents or teachers using an external activating device. The yield from this type of recorder depends on the selectivity of the physician but it can be most useful in children with infrequent major syncope. The recording in Figure 3.1 is from a 4-year-old boy with infrequent syncope. It shows an episode of polymorphic ventricular tachycardia. He was proven to have congenital long QT syndrome.

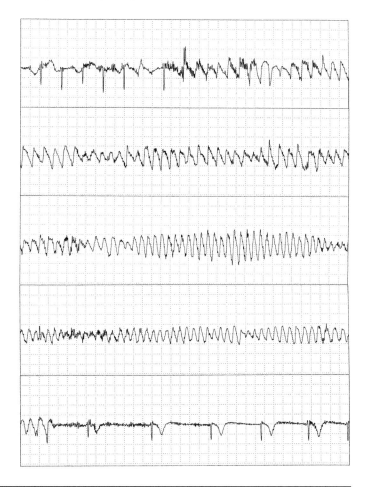

Figure 3.1

Concise Guide to Pediatric Arrhythmias, First Edition. Christopher Wren.
© 2012 John Wiley & Sons, Ltd. Published 2012 by John Wiley & Sons, Ltd.

Transesophageal electrophysiology study

The transesophageal electrophysiology study is not widely employed in pediatric practice because of its limited physical acceptability. It involves peroral or pernasal positioning of a pacing wire in the esophagus behind the left atrium. Pacing in this position can usually capture the atria but requires a higher output stimulator than a normal pacing box. Transesophageal pacing can be used in neonates to overdrive atrial flutter or atrioventricular tachycardia, but its use in older children is limited by discomfort and it often requires general anesthesia. It has been advocated for investigation of children with symptoms of palpitation, elucidation of arrhythmia mechanism if tachycardia is documented on ambulatory ECG monitoring, and "risk assessment" in asymptomatic children with a Wolff–Parkinson–White pattern on the ECG. It is perhaps more widely used in some European countries than in the UK, the USA, or elsewhere.

Tilt test

A head-up tilt test is sometimes used for investigation of children older than 6 years with recurrent syncope or presyncope. Protocols vary but all involve the child lying horizontal for 15–20 min before being passively tilted to an angle of 60–80° for up to 45 min or until the development of symptoms. The ECG and blood pressure are recorded continuously. Fainting or a feeling of faintness is usually accompanied by bradycardia and hypotension, and the child is rapidly returned to the horizontal. Less commonly there is a hypotensive response without bradycardia. The most unusual response is cardioinhibitory with bradycardia or asystole before syncope.

A "positive" test response with passive tilting is observed in 40–50% of children with a good history suggesting neurally mediated syncope (see Chapter 35). The sensitivity is increased by infusion of isoprenaline (isoproterenol) but specificity is reduced. The usefulness of the test is limited by false positives and false negatives, but it can be helpful in management of syncope. Figure 3.2 shows the response after a period of tilting in a 14-year-old girl. She became progressively hypotensive and bradycardic at the onset of symptoms. The heart rate and blood pressure recovered quickly after she was restored to a horizontal position.

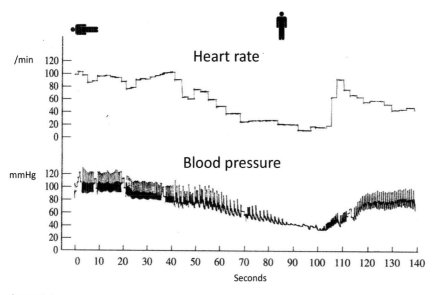

Figure 3.2

Invasive electrophysiology study

This is a large subject and there is space in this text only for a brief review of the indications for its use. In the past electrophysiology studies were performed for a variety of reasons but are now mainly used as part of a catheter ablation procedure (see Chapter 39). The use of electrophysiology study for diagnosis of arrhythmia, assessment of antiarrhythmic drug efficacy, investigation of syncope, and risk assessment is now very limited. It may be helpful in refining the diagnosis in children with suspected or known ventricular tachycardia (see Chapter 18).

The use of electrophysiology study for risk assessment in asymptomatic children with a Wolff–Parkinson–White pattern on the ECG is controversial. Although advocated by some authors, there is little evidence that measurement of the accessory pathway refractory period, or the shortest RR interval in atrial fibrillation, or the inducibility of tachycardia or atrial fibrillation is of any prognostic value. Its usefulness in risk stratification of patients with hypertrophic cardiomyopathy, postoperative tetralogy of Fallot, etc. is unproven.

Key references

Abrams DJ. Invasive electrophysiology in paediatric and congenital heart disease. *Heart* 2007;**93**:383–91.

Brembilla-Perrot B, Groben L, Chometon F, et al. Rapid and low-cost method to prove the nature of no documented tachycardia in children and teenagers without pre-excitation syndrome. *Europace* 2009;**11**:1083–9.

Brignole M, Vardas P, Hoffman E,et al. Indications for the use of diagnostic implantable and external ECG loop recorders. *Europace* 2009;**11**:671–87.

Campbell RM, Strieper MJ, Frias PA, et al. Survey of current practice of pediatric electrophysiologists for asymptomatic Wolff–Parkinson–White syndrome. *Pediatrics* 2003;**111**:e245–7.

Kinlay S, Leitch JW, Neil A, et al. Cardiac event recorders yield more diagnoses and are more cost-effective than 48-hour Holter monitoring in patients with palpitations. A controlled clinical trial. *Ann Intern Med* 1996;**124**:16–20.

Seifer CM, Kenny RA. Head-up tilt testing in children. *Eur Heart J* 2001;**22**:1968–7.

Szili-Torok T, Mikhaylov E, Witsenburg M. Transoesophageal electrophysiology study for children: can we swallow the limitations? *Europace* 2009;**11**:987–8.

Yeung B, McLeod K. The implantable loop recorder in children. *Heart* 2008;**94**:888–91.

4   The normal ECG and variants

Sinus rhythm

In normal sinus rhythm every beat originates in the sinus node. The P wave is generated as atrial depolarization occurs. There is a brief delay from slow conduction in the atrioventricular (AV) node to optimize ventricular filling, shown by the isoelectric PR segment. Electrical conduction to the ventricles occurs at high speed via the His–Purkinje system to allow near-synchronous ventricular contraction, and produces the QRS complex. Ventricular repolarization takes place more slowly and is shown by the T wave. Only after repolarization is complete can the next depolarization occur.

We recognize sinus rhythm on the ECG when the P wave, of normal shape, duration, and axis, is followed, after a normal PR interval, by a QRS complex (Figure 4.1). Every P wave is followed by a QRS and every QRS is preceded by a P wave. We can measure the heart rate, PR interval, QRS duration, and QT interval, among other things (Figure 4.2).

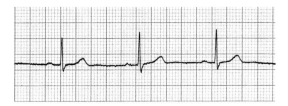

Figure 4.1

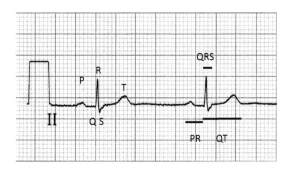

Figure 4.2

Concise Guide to Pediatric Arrhythmias, First Edition. Christopher Wren.
© 2012 John Wiley & Sons, Ltd. Published 2012 by John Wiley & Sons, Ltd.

Heart rate

The sinus rate varies continually within each individual and varies with age. Assessment of whether the heart rate is normal is not possible without knowledge of the patient's age and the circumstances of the recording. Several studies have published normal ECG measurements in children. Figure 4.3 shows the median heart rate (solid line) and 2nd and 98th centiles (dotted lines) for sinus rate in different age groups, and so gives some idea of the range of "normal" heart rate on ECGs recorded at rest.

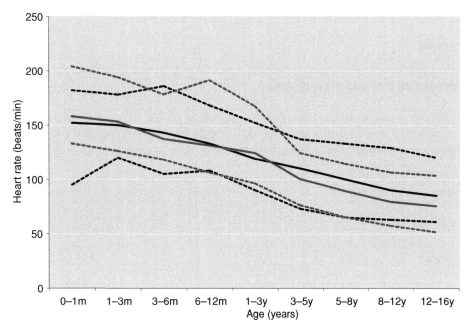

Figure 4.3 Drawn from data published by Davignon et al (1980) (black lines) and Rijnbeek et al (2001) (red lines).

The recording in Figure 4.4 shows sinus rhythm with a rate of 145/min. In infancy this would be normal. When we know that the recording was taken at rest in a 10-year-old boy we realize that the rate is too high. Sustained sinus tachycardia is uncommon but in this case was shown to be due to thyrotoxicosis.

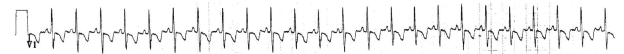

Figure 4.4

This recording in Figure 4.5 is from a sick neonate (with a normal heart) with septicemia and shows a sinus rhythm at 230/min. This is about the maximum possible rate for sinus tachycardia, even in the newborn, and rates above 200/min are rare.

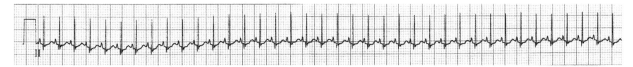

Figure 4.5

QRS duration

The ECG may show a normal or abnormal QRS duration. This measurement is important when we come to analyze the ECG in tachycardia. QRS duration varies with age and QRS complexes are narrower in children than in adults. The median in the newborn is 65 ms with a normal range of 50–80 ms (note how narrow the QRS is in Figure 4.6, from the same infant as in Figure 4.5). In 16 year olds the QRS is 75–115 ms.

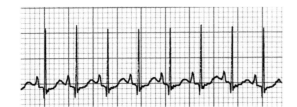

Figure 4.6

Respiratory sinus arrhythmia

Respiratory sinus arrhythmia is an almost universal finding in normal children (Figure 4.7). It describes the phasic variation in sinus rate with acceleration during inspiration and slowing during expiration. It is unusual in infancy.

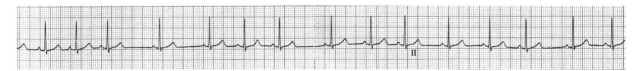

Figure 4.7

Variations in rhythm on ambulatory monitoring

Some minor variations in rhythm on ambulatory monitoring are so common as to be considered normal variants. They include transient Wenckebach AV block during sleep (see Chapter 28) and isolated atrial and ventricular premature beats (see Chapters 11 and 23, respectively).

Notched T waves

Notched T waves in leads V2 and V3 are a common normal finding in normal children (Figure 4.8). The appearance sometimes resembles 2:1 AV block (see Chapter 28) but note that the same appearance is not seen in other leads.

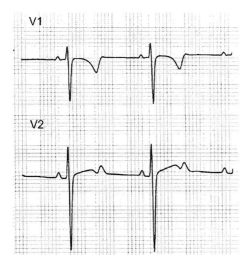

Figure 4.8

Key references

Davignon A, Rautaharju P, Boisselle E, et al. Normal ECG standards for infants and children. *Pediatr Cardiol* 1980;**1**:123–52.

Dickinson DF. The normal ECG in childhood and adolescence. *Heart* 2005;**91**:1626–30.

Garson A. *The Electrocardiogram in Infants and Children: A systematic approach*. Philadelphia: Lea & Febiger, 1983.

Kligfield P, Gettes LS, Bailey JJ, et al. Recommendations for the standardization and interpretation of the electrocardiogram: part I: The electrocardiogram and its technology: a scientific statement from the American Heart Association Electrocardiography and Arrhythmias Committee. *Circulation* 2007;**115**:1306–24.

Rijnbeek PR, Witsenburg M, Schrama E, et al. New normal limits for the paediatric electrocardiogram. *Eur Heart J* 2001;**22**:702–11.

Tipple M. Interpretation of electrocardiograms in infants and children. *Images Paediatr Cardiol* 1999;**1**:3–13. Available at: www.impaedcard.com/issue/issue1/ipc00103.htm (accessed 20 May 2011).

5 Interpretation of the ECG in tachycardia

The management of tachycardia in infants and children depends fundamentally on a precise diagnosis. This will define the mechanism of the arrhythmia, predict the prognosis, and indicate the appropriate treatment.

Much can be learned, as shown below, from careful analysis of the 12-lead ECG in tachycardia and sinus rhythm, as well as a rhythm strip recorded during adenosine administration (see Chapter 6). Other essential pieces of information include the mode of presentation (palpitation, heart failure, syncope, etc.), the current age of the patient, and the age at onset of symptoms.

Sometimes the only ECG traces available are from ambulatory recordings or exercise testing or from an event recorder but these can also provide useful information.

In the past many pediatricians and pediatric cardiologists have been satisfied with deciding whether an arrhythmia is "supraventricular" or ventricular in origin. (Supraventricular tachycardia is one that is not ventricular.) Even if this distinction is made accurately, and that is often not the case, it is an inadequate classification, because there are many types of each of these arrhythmias, each with its own natural history and response to treatment. We should aim, where possible, to define both the substrate and the mechanism of the arrhythmia.

The algorithm in Figure 5.1 shows one method of analyzing the ECG in tachycardia. It is designed to be easy to use and concentrates on analyses that are simple to make (such as whether the QRS is normal or wide, regular or irregular, or resembles right or left bundle branch block, etc.). Less emphasis is placed on interpretations that are sometimes more difficult, such as the timing and relationship of P waves.

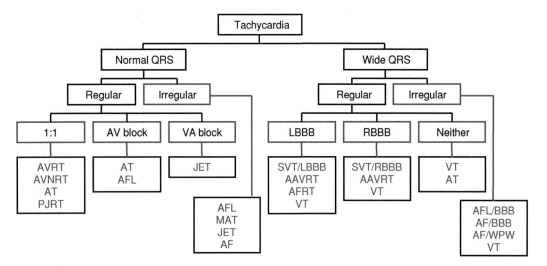

Figure 5.1 AAVRT, antidromic AV re-entry tachycardia; AF, atrial fibrillation; AFL, atrial flutter; AFRT, atriofascicular re-entry tachycardia; AT, atrial tachycardia; AV, atrioventricular; AVNRT, AV nodal re-entry tachycardia; AVRT, AV re-entry tachycardia; BBB, bundle branch block; FAT, focal atrial tachycardia; JET, junctional ectopic tachycardia; MAT, multifocal atrial tachycardia; PJRT, permanent junctional reciprocating tachycardia; SVT, supraventricular tachycardia; VT, ventricular tachycardia; WPW, Wolff–Parkinson–White syndrome.

Concise Guide to Pediatric Arrhythmias, First Edition. Christopher Wren.
© 2012 John Wiley & Sons, Ltd. Published 2012 by John Wiley & Sons, Ltd.

Use of this algorithm will, in most cases, lead to an accurate diagnosis. Each branch of the algorithm in Figure 5.1 leads to a box, outlined in red, which defines a very short differential diagnosis (boxes with red text). Further analysis of the ECG will often pinpoint the precise arrhythmia mechanism, but further information from the patient's age and the response to adenosine is often helpful in distinguishing between arrhythmias within the same box. Each branch of the algorithm, and the subsequent differential diagnosis, are discussed in detail below.

If the tachycardia has a normal QRS and is regular – the most common situation encountered in pediatric practice – it is usually fairly straightforward to decide whether there is one P wave per QRS (a 1:1 relationship) or there are more P waves than QRS complexes (most often 2:1), i.e. tachycardia persists in the face of atrioventricular (AV) block. If the QRS complexes are irregular, P waves or other atrial waves are usually easy to see.

If the tachycardia has a wide QRS and is regular, P waves are more difficult to see and analysis concentrates on the morphology of the QRS complexes, i.e. do they more closely resemble a right or left bundle branch block pattern or neither?

Irregular tachycardias are uncommon in infants and children. Irregularity is defined as a variation in RR interval of 5% or more.

Regular tachycardia with a normal QRS and 1:1 AV relationship

The four types of tachycardia that are regular and have a normal QRS and a 1:1 AV relationship are shown in Figure 5.2. This is by far the most common type of tachycardia ECG encountered in pediatric practice, and is probably what is assumed by pediatricians who arrive at a diagnosis of "supraventricular tachycardia" ("SVT"). We should make note of the rate of tachycardia, and any variations in rate, but the most helpful further analysis is the position or timing of the P wave. The typical P wave positions are shown by red arrows in the examples below.

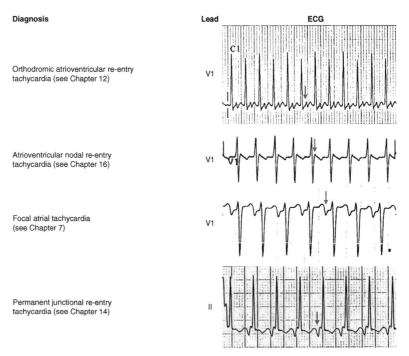

Diagnosis	Lead	ECG
Orthodromic atrioventricular re-entry tachycardia (see Chapter 12)	V1	
Atrioventricular nodal re-entry tachycardia (see Chapter 16)	V1	
Focal atrial tachycardia (see Chapter 7)	V1	
Permanent junctional re-entry tachycardia (see Chapter 14)	II	

Figure 5.2

In *orthodromic AV re-entry tachycardia* (the substrate being an accessory AV pathway – see Chapters 12 and 13), the P wave is usually visible in the first half of the RR interval, often easiest to see in the ST segment in lead V1. In *AV nodal re-entry tachycardia* (see Chapter 16), the P wave is either hidden behind the QRS or, more often, just visible at the end of the QRS – usually easiest to see as a small positive deflection in lead V1. This is a subtle finding and is easiest to confirm by comparing with the QRST morphology in sinus rhythm. These two arrhythmias are common and both have shorter RP than PR intervals – they are known as short RP tachycardias. Both are paroxysmal.

The other two regular tachycardias with normal QRS and a 1:1 AV relationship are long RP tachycardias. They are both usually incessant. *Focal atrial tachycardia* can sometimes be difficult to distinguish from sinus tachycardia (see Chapter 7) because it usually has a normal PR interval. The P wave morphology depends on whether the tachycardia originates in the right or the left atrium. *Permanent junctional re-entry tachycardia* usually has a very long RP interval and is characterized by P waves that are deeply negative in leads II, III, and AVF (see Chapter 14).

The ECG characteristics of these arrhythmias, together with knowledge of the mode of presentation and the age at onset, are usually sufficient to allow us to distinguish between them. If there is doubt about the diagnosis, or if P waves are not visible, administration of adenosine will be helpful (see Chapter 6). Orthodromic AV re-entry tachycardia and AV nodal re-entry tachycardia will stop with adenosine. The ECG in sinus rhythm in the former may be normal or may show pre-excitation. In the latter it will be normal. Adenosine given in atrial ectopic tachycardia usually produces AV block, but the tachycardia continues with a lower ventricular rate. Occasionally tachycardia stops for a few seconds but resumes once the effect of adenosine has worn off. Permanent junctional re-entry tachycardia will stop with adenosine and restart after a few seconds.

Probably the only other arrhythmia that can have a normal QRS and a 1:1 AV relationship is early postoperative junctional tachycardia (see Chapter 31) which can occasionally occur with 1:1 retrograde conduction.

Regular tachycardia with a normal QRS and AV block

A tachycardia that has a normal QRS and exhibits AV block (i.e. there are more P waves than QRS complexes) must originate in the atria. (The only exception to this is AV nodal re-entry tachycardia which can continue with 2:1 AV conduction, but this is really only an observation during electrophysiology testing and is very rarely encountered clinically.)

Tachycardia with AV block usually shows a 2:1 AV relationship, as shown in Figure 5.3, but can show higher grade block, such as 4:1, or variable block such as 3:2 Wenckebach conduction (although in this last case the QRS complexes will be irregular). In the two examples in Figure 5.3, it is fairly easy to see the 2:1 AV relationship. In *atrial tachycardia* there are distinct P waves with an isoelectric interval between them, whereas *atrial flutter* shows a typical saw-tooth appearance with continuous electrical activity.

Diagnosis	Lead	ECG

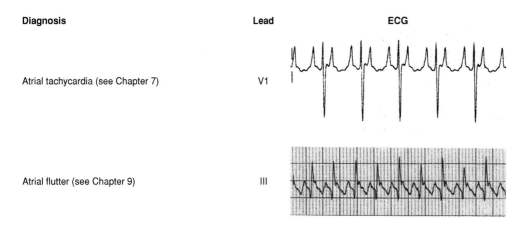

Atrial tachycardia (see Chapter 7)	V1	
Atrial flutter (see Chapter 9)	III	

Figure 5.3

Sometimes it is difficult to tell that 2:1 conduction is present, in which case adenosine is very helpful (see Chapter 6).

Irregular tachycardia with a normal QRS

Tachycardias with normal but irregular QRS complexes are uncommon in pediatric practice. The differential diagnosis is shown in Figure 5.4. Each of these arrhythmias is discussed in detail elsewhere but it is worth noting the rarity of pediatric atrial fibrillation.

Diagnosis	Lead	ECG

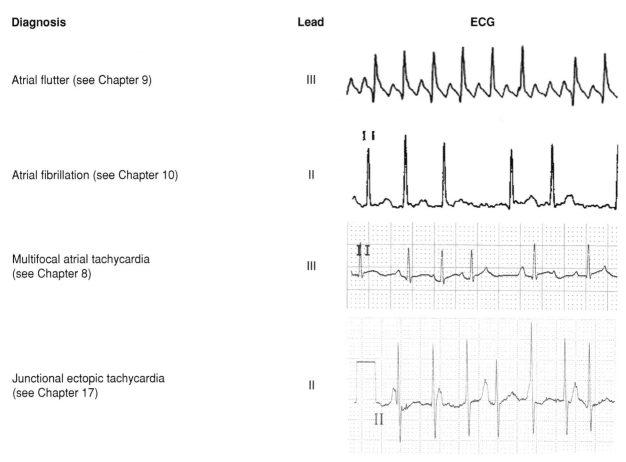

Atrial flutter (see Chapter 9)	III	
Atrial fibrillation (see Chapter 10)	II	
Multifocal atrial tachycardia (see Chapter 8)	III	
Junctional ectopic tachycardia (see Chapter 17)	II	

Figure 5.4

As outlined in the algorithm in Figure 5.1, a different approach is adopted to analysis of tachycardias with a wide QRS. It is best to consider the morphology and regularity of the QRS complexes before looking for P waves, which can be difficult to see. Having said that, if dissociated P waves are obvious, the diagnosis is clearly ventricular tachycardia (see Chapter 18).

QRS analysis in wide complex tachycardia assesses whether the pattern more closely resembles right or left bundle branch block or neither. Before we look at examples of wide QRS tachycardia it is worth considering causes of QRS widening in other situations.

The pattern we recognize as *right bundle branch block* occurs when there is normal rapid conduction in the left bundle but not in the right. As a result depolarization of the right ventricle occurs by slower myocyte-to-myocyte conduction and right ventricular activation is late compared with the left. A similar (but not identical) appearance might be expected if left ventricular activation is earlier than normal. This can occur with either ventricular pre-excitation via a left-sided accessory pathway in Wolff–Parkinson–White syndrome or left ventricular pacing. Examples of these two appearances are compared with right bundle branch block in Figure 5.5 and the similarities are obvious. For clarity only leads V1 and V6 are shown.

Appreciation of the causes of these similarities will be helpful when we come to analyze tachycardias with a right bundle branch block appearance.

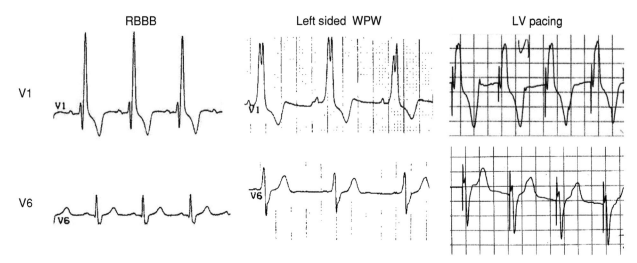

Figure 5.5 RBBB, right bundle branch block; WPW, Wolff–Parkinson–White syndrome.

In a similar way *left bundle branch block* occurs when there is normal conduction in the right bundle but not in the left. Activation of the left ventricle is late compared with the right. We can predict that a similar appearance will be seen if right ventricular activation is earlier than normal – with either ventricular pre-excitation via a right-sided accessory pathway or right ventricular pacing. These two appearances are compared with left bundle branch block in Figure 5.6 and again the similarities are clear.

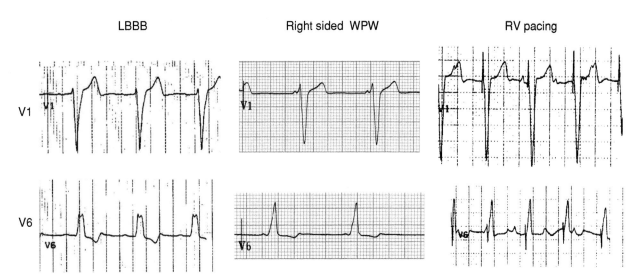

Figure 5.6 LBBB, left bundle branch block; WPW, Wolff–Parkinson–White syndrome.

Regular tachycardia with a wide QRS with right bundle branch block morphology

There are three main possible causes of tachycardia with QRS showing a right bundle branch block (RBBB) appearance (Figure 5.7). Probably the most common in infants and children is *supraventricular tachycardia with rate-related RBBB*, i.e. a tachycardia that would most often have a normal QRS (so usually either AV re-entry tachycardia or AV nodal re-entry) but that produces rate-related block in the right bundle branch, known as functional aberration. Occasionally this appearance is produced by pre-existing RBBB, in other words the QRS is normal for that patient. With aberration or pre-existing RBBB, the second R wave in lead V1 is taller, as in the first example in Figure 5.7. Sometimes the aberration is transient, and the QRS reverts to normal after a few beats but tachycardia continues. When sinus rhythm is restored the ECG may be normal or show RBBB, or be pre-excited (which will prove the existence of an accessory pathway).

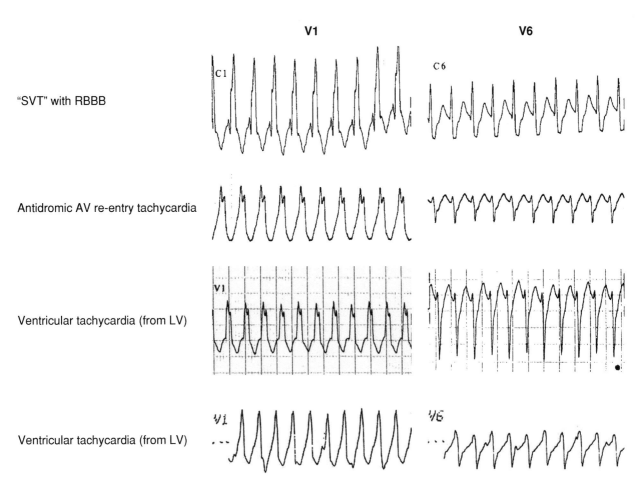

V1

V6

"SVT" with RBBB

Antidromic AV re-entry tachycardia

Ventricular tachycardia (from LV)

Ventricular tachycardia (from LV)

Figure 5.7 AV, atrioventricular; LV, left ventricle; RBBB, right bundle branch block; SVT, supraventricular tachycardia.

Much less common is *antidromic re-entry tachycardia* in Wolff–Parkinson–White syndrome (see Chapter 13). This produces a maximally pre-excited QRS, effectively a giant delta wave. As shown in the second example in Figure 5.7, the first R wave in V1 is taller. When sinus rhythm is restored the ECG will show pre-excitation with a pattern predicting a left-sided pathway.

The third possible diagnosis is *ventricular tachycardia*, and two examples are shown in Figure 5.7. We can deduce from the RBBB-like pattern that the tachycardia originates in the left ventricle. Again the first R wave in V1 is usually taller. Ventricular tachycardia will be confirmed beyond any doubt if dissociated P waves are seen, as in the fourth example below. The two examples of left ventricular tachycardia shown differ in the speed of the upstroke in the R wave (the ventricular activation time). This presumably results from the relationship of the point of origin of the tachycardia to the specialized conduction system – the closer it is the faster the R wave upstroke. When sinus rhythm is restored the ECG will probably be normal but may show changes relating to the cause of the tachycardia or resulting from the effects of any drugs administered (such as QT prolongation with amiodarone or QRS prolongation with flecainide).

Regular tachycardia with a wide QRS with left bundle branch block morphology

Four different arrhythmias may produce a regular tachycardia with an appearance similar to left bundle branch block (LBBB). Perhaps the most common in pediatric practice is tachycardia which would otherwise have a normal QRS but causes functional aberration, i.e. some form of *supraventricular tachycardia with rate-related LBBB*. In the first example in Figure 5.8, note that the onset of the QRS is very sharp. LBBB aberration may be transient at the onset of tachycardia or persist. As a sustained appearance it is perhaps more common than RBBB aberration, especially in infants. Once sinus rhythm is restored the ECG may be normal, or show LBBB or show pre-excitation.

V1   V6

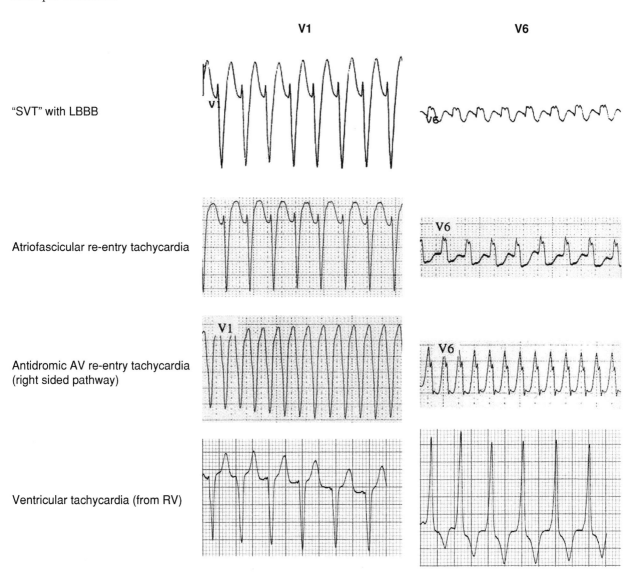

"SVT" with LBBB

Atriofascicular re-entry tachycardia

Antidromic AV re-entry tachycardia (right sided pathway)

Ventricular tachycardia (from RV)

Figure 5.8 AV, atrioventricular; LBBB, left bundle branch block; RV, right ventricle; SVT, supraventricular tachycardia.

Atriofascicular re-entry tachycardia is a rare arrhythmia seen in older children (see Chapter 15). It always causes permanent LBBB appearance during tachycardia and is indistinguishable from SVT with rate-related LBBB on a single recording – as in the second example in Figure 5.8. It is suspected especially if ECGs from multiple episodes of tachycardia all show LBBB. Atriofascicular re-entry will stop with intravenous adenosine and the ECG will then be normal in sinus rhythm.

Antidromic AV re-entry tachycardia is rare but occurs more often with right- than left-sided pathways (see Chapter 13). The third example in Figure 5.8 shows a very rapid tachycardia with a slow onset to the S wave in V1 and R wave in V6, which is a large delta wave. Antidromic AV re-entry will usually stop with adenosine (there are rare exceptions if the re-entry circuit involves two pathways) and the ECG will then show ventricular pre-excitation.

A similar appearance is seen in *ventricular tachycardia* originating in the right ventricle (see Chapter 22). The exact morphology of the QRS will vary with the type of ventricular tachycardia.

Regular tachycardia with a wide QRS and neither RBBB nor LBBB morphology

Sometimes the ECG shows a sinusoidal appearance that does not really resemble either RBBB or LBBB. The diagnosis is usually *ventricular tachycardia*, as in the first example in Figure 5.9. Just about the only other arrhythmia that may occasionally produce a similar effect is *atrial flutter* or *atrial tachycardia with 1:1 AV conduction*, usually with some superadded drug effect on the QRS. The second example in Figure 5.9 is from a neonate born to a mother who had been treated with flecainide for fetal "SVT."

Diagnosis	Lead	ECG
Ventricular tachycardia	V1	
Atrial flutter with BBB (especially drug effect)	V1	

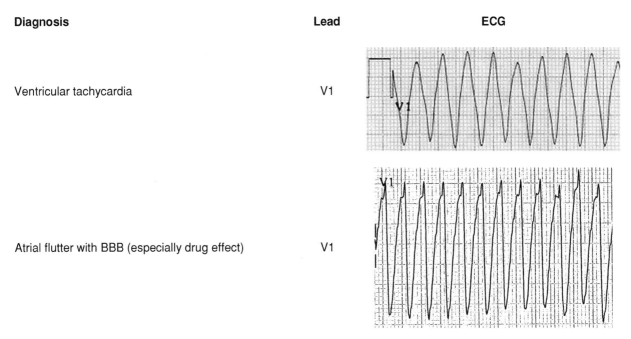

Figure 5.9 BBB, bundle branch block.

Irregular tachycardia with a wide QRS

This type of arrhythmia is rare in children. The first two examples in Figure 5.10 show atrial fibrillation in which the QRS complexes are characteristically irregularly irregular (see Chapter 10). The first recording in Figure 5.10 shows *atrial fibrillation with LBBB* in a teenager with dilated cardiomyopathy. The second shows *atrial fibrillation with ventricular pre-excitation* in Wolff–Parkinson–White syndrome (see Chapter 13). The irregularity can be difficult to see if the ventricular rate is very high but becomes more noticeable at slightly lower rates. Note that in both these example the QRS morphology is constant. This contrasts with the third recording, which shows *polymorphic ventricular tachycardia* in which the QRS axis is constantly changing. Otherwise known as torsades de pointes, this tachycardia is usually seen in long QT syndrome (see Chapter 25). It causes syncope and is, therefore, usually documented only on some kind of ECG monitor or ambulatory recording.

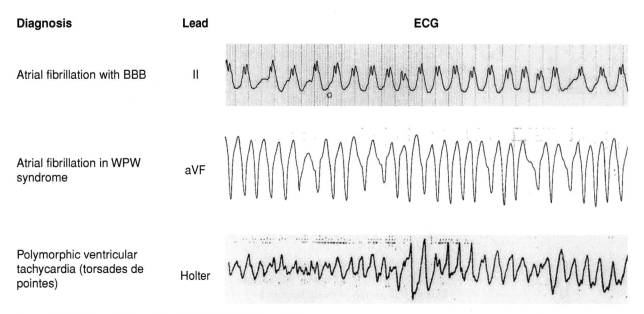

Diagnosis	Lead	ECG
Atrial fibrillation with BBB	II	
Atrial fibrillation in WPW syndrome	aVF	
Polymorphic ventricular tachycardia (torsades de pointes)	Holter	

Figure 5.10 BBB, bundle branch block; WPW, Wolff–Parkinson–White.

Changing QRS morphology in tachycardia

It is not uncommon to see a wide QRS for two or three beats at the onset of tachycardia which then reverts to normal after a few beats, but these are not premature ventricular beats. The refractory periods of all cardiac tissues vary with rate and either the left or right bundle may be temporarily refractory after a sudden increase in rate, as shown in Figure 5.11.

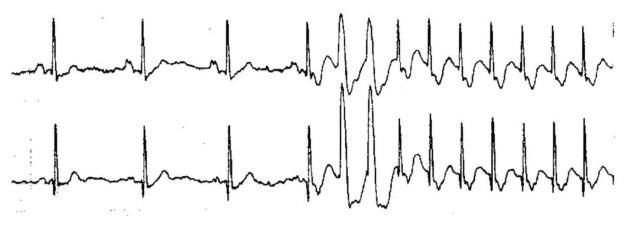

Figure 5.11

If the tachycardia is caused by AV re-entry via an accessory pathway, the tachycardia is sometimes seen to speed up as the bundle branch block resolves (this is discussed further in Chapter 12). From this we can conclude that the pathway is on the same side of the heart as the bundle branch block. Resolution of functional block in the opposite bundle branch will have no effect on rate, as in the example above.

Changing QRS morphology during tachycardia is occasionally seen in other clinical situations. Bidirectional ventricular tachycardia is the characteristic arrhythmia in catecholaminergic polymorphic ventricular tachycardia (see Chapter 26). The QRS complexes alternate but also change over time, as shown in Figure 5.12.

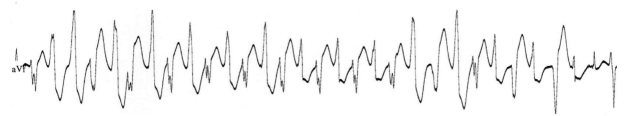

Figure 5.12

Key references

Dendi R, Josephson ME. A new algorithm in the differential diagnosis of wide complex tachycardia. *Eur Heart J* 2007;**28**:525–6.

Fox DJ, Tischenko A, Krahn AD, et al. Supraventricular tachycardia: diagnosis and management. *Mayo Clin Proc* 2008;**83**:1400–11.

Jaeggi ET, Gilljam T, Bauersfeld U, et al. Electrocardiographic differentiation of typical atrioventricular node reentrant tachycardia from atrioventricular reciprocating tachycardia mediated by concealed accessory pathway in children. *Am J Cardiol* 2003;**91**:1084–9.

Kistler PM, Roberts-Thomson KC, Haqqani HM, et al. P-wave morphology in focal atrial tachycardia: development of an algorithm to predict the anatomic site of origin. *J Am Coll Cardiol* 2006;**48**:1010–17.

Vereckei A, Duray G, Szénási G, et al. Application of a new algorithm in the differential diagnosis of wide QRS complex tachycardia. *Eur Heart J* 2007;**28**:589–600.

Wellens HJ. The value of the ECG in the diagnosis of supraventricular tachycardias. *Eur Heart J* 1996;**17**(suppl C):10–20.

Wellens HJJ. Electrophysiology: Ventricular tachycardia: diagnosis of broad QRS complex tachycardia. *Heart* 2001;**86**:579–85.

Wren C. Incessant tachycardias. *Eur Heart J* 1998;**19**(suppl E):E32–6, E54–9.

Adenosine in the diagnosis of tachycardias

Intravenous adenosine is the first-line treatment for any sustained regular tachycardia in infancy or childhood, with either a normal or a wide QRS. The main aim is termination of tachycardia but any change in the ECG, even if only transient, may give useful diagnostic information.

Adenosine is not recommended for sustained *irregular* tachycardias, partly because the mechanism of the arrhythmia should already be apparent from analysis of the ECG (see Chapter 5) and partly because there is the possibility of producing hemodynamic deterioration from acceleration of the ventricular rate (see Chapter 37).

The initial dose of adenosine is $100\,\mu g/kg$ in children or $150\,\mu g/kg$ in infants. It is very important to record the ECG during administration (preferably three leads – I, aVF, and V1) as well as a 12-lead ECG before and after. It is not adequate simply to observe the ECG on a monitor because termination of tachycardia, even for only one beat, will prove the efficacy of the drug and provide important diagnostic information (see below). If the first dose is ineffective, the second should be 50 or $100\,\mu g/kg$ higher (see Chapter 37).

The clinical use of adenosine takes advantage of its dominant effect of slowing atrioventricular (AV) conduction. Many common types of "supraventricular" tachycardia involve re-entry through the AV node. Such arrhythmias are reliably terminated by adenosine, because they cannot continue in the presence of AV nodal block.

Less common re-entry tachycardias (such as permanent junctional reciprocating tachycardia or atriofascicular re-entry tachycardia) are usually terminated, if only transiently. The effect of adenosine on atrial arrhythmias is less predictable. It will not terminate atrial flutter but does slow AV conduction to unmask the flutter. This can be a great help in diagnosis if 1:1 or 2:1 AV conduction makes precise diagnosis difficult. The effect on other atrial arrhythmias varies. Focal atrial tachycardia may be unmasked by showing 2:1 conduction but may also be transiently suppressed, making differential diagnosis from sinus tachycardia more difficult (see Chapter 7). Adenosine rarely terminates ventricular tachycardia, but careful analysis of the ECG during administration may identify production of retrograde block.

Diagnostic use of adenosine

Tachycardias may respond to administration of adenosine in a number of ways. The response will be a significant help in assessment of the mechanism of the tachycardia. Possible effects of adenosine are shown below, along with the arrhythmias that are likely to show that effect.

Tachycardia stops

This is the most likely response if a sufficient dose has been given. It is seen most commonly in AV re-entry tachycardia and in AV nodal re-entry. It is worth looking to see if tachycardia stops with AV block – the most common response – shown by a

Concise Guide to Pediatric Arrhythmias, First Edition. Christopher Wren.
© 2012 John Wiley & Sons, Ltd. Published 2012 by John Wiley & Sons, Ltd.

non-conducted P wave (black arrow in Figure 6.1). Note also the obvious ventricular pre-excitation in sinus rhythm (red arrow), confirming the presence of an accessory pathway.

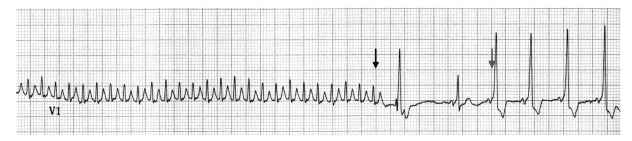

Figure 6.1

Sometimes tachycardia stops with retrograde block – shown by a missing P wave in Figure 6.2 (arrow). This may also be seen in permanent junctional reciprocating tachycardia (see Chapter 14) or in other rare forms of tachycardia such as antidromic AV re-entry tachycardia (see Chapter 13) or atriofascicular re-entry (see Chapter 15).

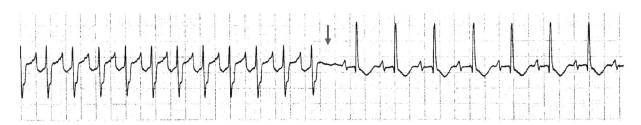

Figure 6.2

Tachycardia stops transiently and then restarts

This may be seen in AV re-entry tachycardia (Figure 6.3), and in rarer forms of AV re-entry such as permanent junctional reciprocating tachycardia (see Chapter 14).

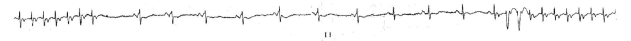

Figure 6.3

Tachycardia slows transiently and then speeds up

This may be seen in sinus tachycardia (Figure 6.4) and sometimes in atrial tachycardia.

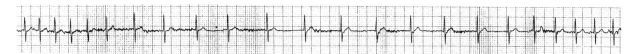

Figure 6.4

Tachycardia continues in the presence of AV block

This confirms atrial tachycardia or atrial flutter. In Figure 6.5, focal atrial tachycardia, the atrial rate is unchanged but conduction is reduced from 1:1 to 2:1, proving the diagnosis.

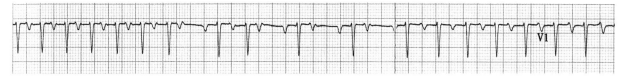

Figure 6.5

In Figure 6.6 the rhythm is initially atrial flutter with 2:1 conduction but flutter waves are not easy to see. The effect of adenosine on the AV node reduces conduction to 4:1, making the diagnosis obvious.

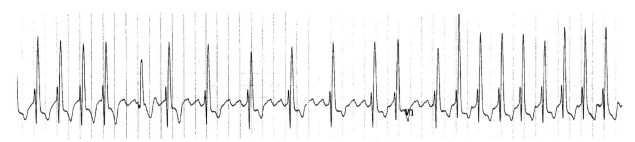

Figure 6.6

Tachycardia continues in the presence of ventriculoatrial block

This requires careful analysis to identify but will confirm the presence of ventricular tachycardia (Figure 6.7) or junctional ectopic tachycardia (see Chapters 17 and 31). At the start of the trace in Figure 6.7 there is 1:1 retrograde conduction (red arrows show retrogradely conducted P waves). Adenosine causes retrograde block, which allows a sinus capture beat (a sinus P wave produces a conducted sinus beat with a normal QRS) followed by obviously dissociated P waves (black arrows).

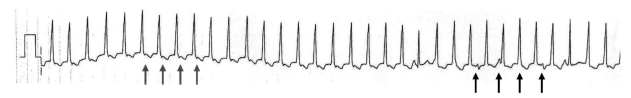

Figure 6.7

Other findings

In Figure 6.8, tachycardia breaks transiently, ending with a non-conducted P wave (red arrow). The two sinus beats are each followed by a P wave of the same morphology as the P wave in tachycardia (black arrow). This appearance is not uncommon and is characteristic of AV re-entry with an accessory pathway. Tachycardia restarts after the third sinus beat.

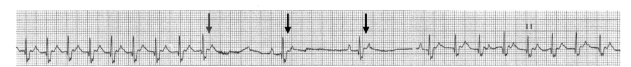

Figure 6.8

Key references

Dixon J, Foster K, Wyllie J, Wren C. Guidelines and adenosine dosing for supraventricular tachycardia. *Arch Dis Child* 2005;**90**:1190–1.

Glatter KA, Cheng J, Dorostkar P, *et al.* Electrophysiologic effects of adenosine in patients with supraventricular tachycardia. *Circulation* 1999;**99**:1034–40.

Wren C. Adenosine in paediatric arrhythmias. *Paediatr Perinat Drug Ther* 2006;**7**:114–17.

7 Atrial tachycardia

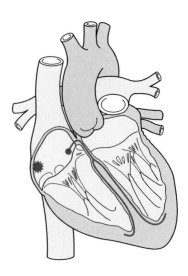

There are many different types of atrial tachycardia. All have in common the feature that they do not require participation of the atrioventricular (AV) node, or the sinus node, or the ventricles for maintenance of tachycardia. Atrial tachycardia is, therefore, unaffected by AV block, either spontaneous or adenosine induced. The definition also excludes other types of atrial arrhythmia such as atrial fibrillation and atrial flutter (macro re-entry).

The terminology of atrial tachycardias has been confusing. In previous years the term "atrial tachycardia" was sometimes used synonymously with supraventricular tachycardia, particularly in North America, but that terminology is now outdated.

The label focal atrial tachycardia has been used recently to describe atrial arrhythmias that originate from a point source or localized area of the atrium. Such arrhythmias have also been known as atrial ectopic tachycardia and ectopic atrial tachycardia. The term "focal atrial tachycardia" does not imply a mechanism, which may be micro re-entry, automaticity, or triggered activity, although abnormal automaticity (as in atrial ectopic tachycardia) is the most likely.

Other atrial arrhythmias – atrial flutter (see Chapter 9), multifocal atrial tachycardia (see Chapter 8), late postoperative atrial tachycardia (see Chapter 32), and atrial fibrillation (see Chapter 10) – are discussed elsewhere.

Presentation and natural history of atrial tachycardia

Atrial tachycardia may present at any age. It is a less common cause of tachycardia in the fetus but is seen in newborn babies and in infancy. In children atrial tachycardia tends to be an incessant arrhythmia and does not usually cause palpitations. More typically it presents with a tachycardia-induced cardiomyopathy in a child with no awareness of tachycardia. There is usually only a short history of being unwell, with lethargy, breathlessness, and vomiting. The natural history depends on the age at diagnosis. In infants there is a high rate of spontaneous resolution so drug treatment is usually appropriate. In older children tachycardia usually persists and catheter ablation is the preferred treatment.

Concise Guide to Pediatric Arrhythmias, First Edition. Christopher Wren.
© 2012 John Wiley & Sons, Ltd. Published 2012 by John Wiley & Sons, Ltd.

ECG diagnosis of atrial tachycardia

Atrial tachycardia is usually frequent or incessant so documentation on ECG is generally fairly straightforward. The rate varies considerably between patients, being as high as 300/min in some infants but generally in the range 150–250/min in children. The ECG typically shows distinct P waves with an isoelectric interval between them. Each P wave is followed by a QRS with a PR interval that may be normal or slightly prolonged. The main differential diagnosis of atrial tachycardia is sinus tachycardia; it can sometimes be difficult to distinguish the two in a child presenting with a cardiomyopathy.

In atrial tachycardia the rate shows considerable variability, with abrupt rate changes and occasional non-conducted beats, and the P wave morphology is often abnormal. The P wave shape depends on the anatomical site of origin of the tachycardia. The ECG in Figure 7.1 comes from a 5-year-old boy who presented acutely with severe heart failure. It shows a rate of around 170/min with a normal frontal P wave axis and negative P waves in lead V1. At electrophysiological investigation this was shown to be a focal tachycardia on the anterior right atrial wall.

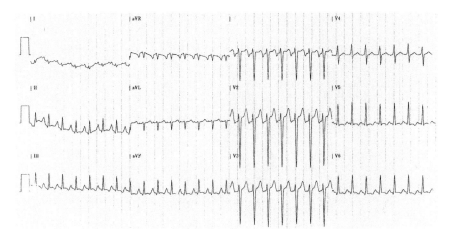

Figure 7.1

Figure 7.2 comes from an 11-year-old boy with a left atrial tachycardia that had an origin close to the left lower pulmonary vein. He also presented with heart failure and his ECG shows a rate of 170/min with P waves that are negative in leads I, II, and V6, and positive in V1.

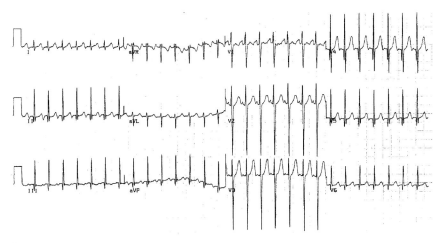

Figure 7.2

If the diagnosis is not clear from the 12-lead ECG, further observation of the ECG may help. Some infants and children with atrial tachycardia exhibit occasional non-conducted beats, something that is not seen in sinus tachycardia or in AV re-entry tachycardia. Figure 7.3 comes from a neonate with sustained tachycardia at just over 300/min. Unlike the more commonly seen AV re-entry tachycardia, this ECG shows occasional irregularity due to non-conducted P waves. The PR interval is long and most of the P waves occur just after the previous QRS (red arrows). The PR interval after the pause is normal but all the P waves are the same shape.

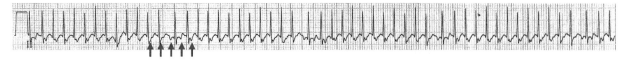

Figure 7.3

Figure 7.4, from an older child, shows the same phenomenon, although the P waves are a little less easy to see (black arrows). Again the PR interval after the pause is shorter but it prolongs over a couple of beats.

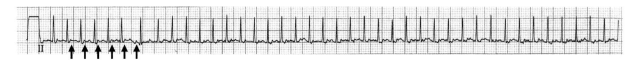

Figure 7.4

In Figure 7.5, from a 14-year-old boy with unoperated, congenitally corrected transposition of the great arteries, there is an atrial rate of around 240/min (arrows) with 4:3 AV Wenckebach conduction, so the QRS complexes are irregular and occur in groups of three.

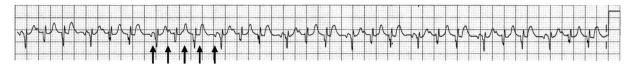

Figure 7.5

In all three examples above, the spontaneous AV block excludes the possibility of AV nodal re-entry or AV re-entry with an accessory pathway. If AV block is not seen, administration of adenosine is usually helpful. Figure 7.6 below shows the response to adenosine in a 5-year-old boy with sustained tachycardia. The atrial tachycardia is unaffected as conduction drops to 2:1. As the adenosine effect wears off there is transient 3:2 conduction before 1:1 conduction resumes.

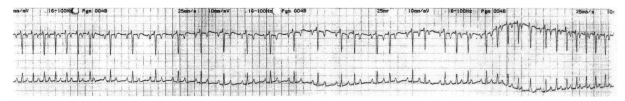

Figure 7.6

Figure 7.7 is another example of adenosine administration in a 10-year-old boy. Again there is transient AV block with no effect on the atrial rate or P wave morphology.

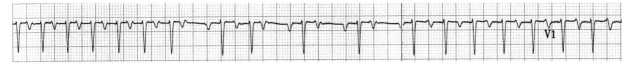

Figure 7.7

However, adenosine will sometimes temporarily suppress atrial tachycardia so transient restoration of sinus rhythm does not exclude the diagnosis. In Figure 7.8, another rhythm strip from the same child as in Figure 7.7, adenosine stops the tachycardia briefly. Tachycardia P waves are negative in lead V1, showing the anterior right atrial origin of the arrhythmia (black arrows). The sinus P waves are similar but have a different shape (red arrows). Tachycardia resumes as soon as the effect of the adenosine wears off.

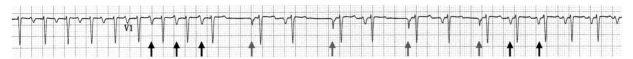

Figure 7.8

Figure 7.9 shows another example of adenosine suppression of atrial tachycardia, this time in a young infant. The sinus P wave (red arrow) has a different shape to those in tachycardia (black arrows).

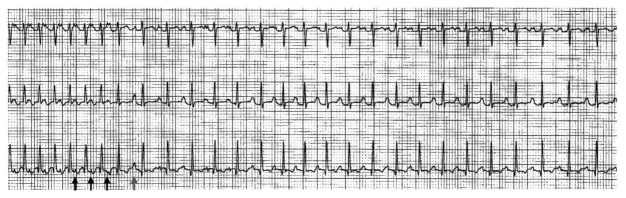

Figure 7.9

As the adenosine effect wears off a few seconds later, tachycardia restarts (Figure 7.10) – notice again the change in P wave shape (red arrows). This rhythm strip also shows another characteristic of atrial tachycardia, that of "warm up." The rate gradually increases over the first several beats – one of the typical features of arrhythmias caused by increased automaticity.

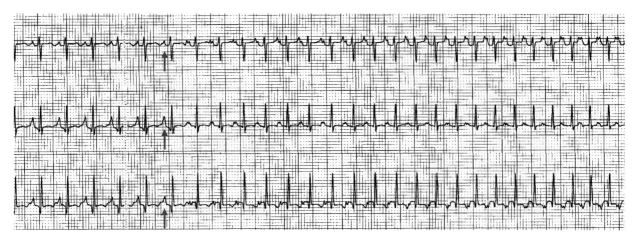

Figure 7.10

Figure 7.11 shows a final example of adenosine administration in atrial tachycardia. Here we see the production of AV block, sometimes briefly 2:1 conduction but also variable AV Wenckebach conduction.

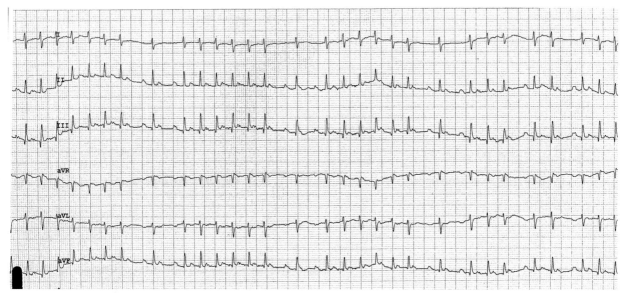

Figure 7.11

Treatment of atrial tachycardia

As mentioned above, there is usually a different management plan for infants and young children than for older children. Medication is the preferred option in infants and small children. Digoxin is ineffective and the drugs most likely to achieve rate and rhythm control are amiodarone and flecainide, sometimes with the addition of a β-blocker. Medication can often be withdrawn without recurrence of tachycardia after 12 or 24 months.

Spontaneous resolution of tachycardia is less likely in older children. In those who present with a sustained arrhythmia and poor ventricular function, the best option may be an urgent electrophysiology study with tachycardia mapping and radiofrequency ablation, if facilities are available. An alternative plan is short-term drug treatment, with either amiodarone or a drug such as flecainide. This will allow the clinical situation to stabilize, and ventricular function to improve, before later ablation. However, tachycardia does not necessarily reappear immediately after drug treatment is stopped so patience and flexibility may be required in the scheduling of the ablation procedure.

The results of ablation are good, with a high success rate and low risk of recurrence. Experience has shown that the most common sites of origin of the tachycardia are the appendage and crista terminalis in the right atrium and the appendage or close to the origins of the pulmonary veins in the left atrium.

Key references

Cummings RM, Mahle WT, Streiper MJ, et al. Outcomes following electroanatomic mapping and ablation for the treatment of ectopic atrial tachycardia in the pediatric population. *Pediatr Cardiol* 2008;**29**:393–7.

Gelb BD, Garson A Jr. Noninvasive discrimination of right atrial ectopic tachycardia from sinus tachycardia in "dilated cardiomyopathy." *Am Heart J* 1990;**120**:886–91.

Kistler PM, Roberts-Thomson KC, Haqqani HM, et al. P-wave morphology in focal atrial tachycardia: development of an algorithm to predict the anatomic site of origin. *J Am Coll Cardiol* 2006;**48**:1010–17.

Rosso R, Kistler P. Focal atrial tachycardia. *Heart* 2010;**96**:181–5.

Salerno J, Kertesz N, Friedman R, et al. Clinical course of atrial ectopic tachycardia is age-dependent: results and treatment in children <3 or ≥3 years of age. *J Am Coll Cardiol* 2004;**43**:438–44.

Saoudi N, Cosio F, Waldo A, et al. A classification of atrial flutter and regular atrial tachycardia according to electrophysiological mechanisms and anatomical bases; a statement from a Joint Expert Group from the Working Group of Arrhythmias of the European Society of Cardiology and the North American Society of Pacing and Electrophysiology. *Eur Heart J* 2001;**22**:1162–82.

Seslar SP, Alexander ME, Berul CI, et al. Ablation of nonautomatic focal atrial tachycardia in children and adults with congenital heart disease. *J Cardiovasc Electrophysiol* 2006;**17**:359–65.

Multifocal atrial tachycardia

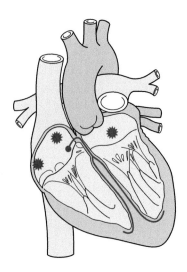

Multifocal atrial tachycardia (also known as chaotic atrial tachycardia) is an uncommon arrhythmia seen in neonates or in early infancy. It is characterized by multiple P waves with varying P wave morphology. Often many of the P waves are not conducted so the ventricular rhythm is irregular and the rate may be more or less normal, or even a little slow. Multifocal atrial tachycardia is often an incidental finding during evaluation for minor illness or it may be noted during neonatal examination. Less commonly the ventricular rate is persistently high and this may cause severe ventricular impairment and heart failure.

ECG diagnosis

To be confident of the diagnosis we expect to see a tachycardia with at least three different shaped P waves and variable PP intervals as shown in Figure 8.1 (arrows).

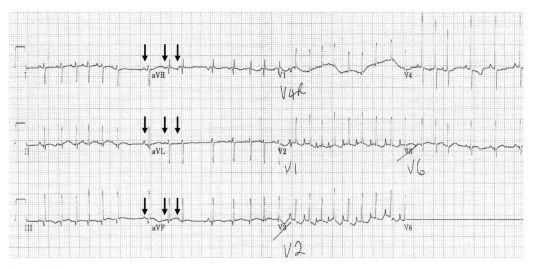

Figure 8.1

Concise Guide to Pediatric Arrhythmias, First Edition. Christopher Wren.
© 2012 John Wiley & Sons, Ltd. Published 2012 by John Wiley & Sons, Ltd.

CHAPTER 8 Multifocal atrial tachycardia

The PR interval varies with different origins of the P waves. There is usually variable atrioventricular (AV) block. Most QRS complexes are normal but some, with short RR intervals, show aberrancy (i.e. they have a rate-related bundle branch block).

In Figure 8.2 three different P wave shapes can be seen (black arrows). Note that some P waves are not conducted (red arrows) and that the PP interval is irregular.

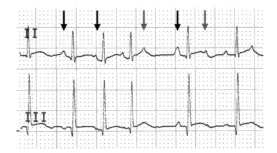

Figure 8.2

The PP intervals are usually isoelectric but occasionally an appearance similar to coarse atrial fibrillation is seen. In Figure 8.3 the P waves are very rapid and irregular and look almost like atrial fibrillation. Few of the P waves are conducted so the ventricular rate is a little slow and irregular.

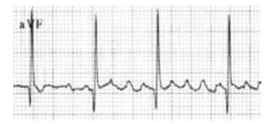

Figure 8.3

In Figure 8.4 the P waves are rapid and irregular, mimicking atrial fibrillation or even flutter, but again there are multiple P wave morphologies and irregular PP intervals.

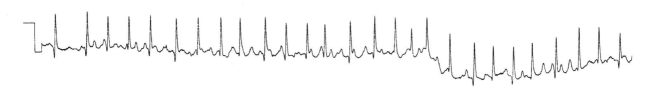

Figure 8.4

In Figure 8.5 some of the QRS complexes are wide. All are preceded by P waves so these are not ventricular premature beats. The wide QRS complexes follow the short RR intervals so this is aberrant conduction. As seen in the rhythm strip at the bottom, QRS complexes with both right and left bundle branch block occur.

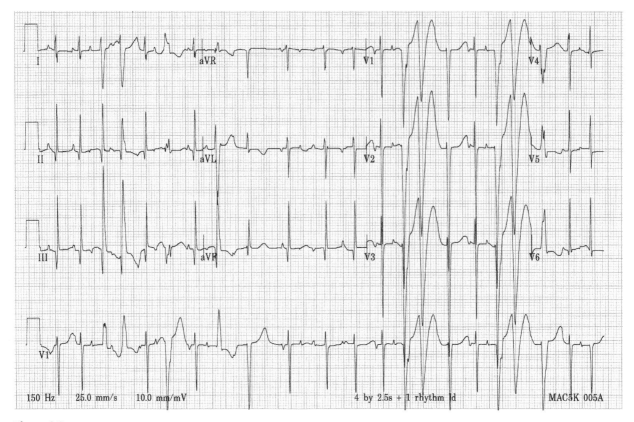

Figure 8.5

Adenosine is not a great help in reaching a diagnosis in multifocal atrial tachycardia. The diagnosis is usually obvious from the ECG as discussed above. Adenosine may transiently suppress the abnormal P waves to restore sinus rhythm for a few seconds.

Treatment

If the ventricular rate is relatively normal and the infant is asymptomatic with normal heart function, it may well be that no treatment is required. Cardioversion is unsuccessful, not surprisingly because the arrhythmia is effectively restarting all the time. A β-blocker is probably the drug of choice, with an occasional patient with poor ventricular function needing treatment with amiodarone.

The natural history of multifocal atrial tachycardia is spontaneous resolution in weeks or a few months. In those who require drug treatment, medication can be withdrawn after that time. The long-term outlook is excellent, with no late recurrence.

Key references

Bradley DJ, Fischbach PS, Law IH, et al. The clinical course of multifocal atrial tachycardia in infants and children. *J Am Coll Cardiol* 2001;**38**:401–8.

Dodo H, Gow RM, Hamilton RM, et al. Chaotic atrial rhythm in children. *Am Heart J* 1995; **129**:990–5.

Fish FA, Mehta AV, Johns JA. Characteristics and management of chaotic atrial tachycardia of infancy. *Am J Cardiol* 1996;**78**:1052–5.

Salim MA, Case CL, Gillette PC. Chaotic atrial tachycardia in children. *Am Heart J* 1995; **129**:831–3.

9   Atrial flutter

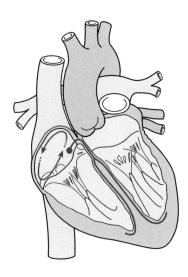

Atrial flutter occurs in two main clinical situations in pediatric practice – in neonates with structurally normal hearts and in children with structural heart disease or impaired cardiac function. It also occurs in adults with congenital heart defects late after surgical repair (see Chapter 32).

Atrial flutter is produced by macro re-entry in the right atrium. In the common, so-called typical or counterclockwise atrial flutter, there is a wave of depolarization travelling up the atrial septum, down the lateral atrial wall, and through the isthmus (between the tricuspid valve and the inferior vena cava).

Atrial flutter is recognized on the ECG by continuous electrical activity in the atria, as shown by flutter waves which produce a "sawtooth" pattern, typically best seen in leads II, III, and aVF. Atrial flutter is distinguished from atrial tachycardia, in which there is an isoelectric period between P waves, although in reality there may overlap between the two, especially late after open cardiac surgery.

The atrial rate varies between patients but is often around 440/min in newborn babies and around 300/min in older children. It may be even slower in late post-operative patients, such as after a classic Fontan operation (see Chapter 32). In the example in Figure 9.1, from a neonate, the atrial rate is around 460/min, which with 2:1 atrioventricular (AV) conduction gives a ventricular rate of around 230/min. The flutter waves are easily seen in inferior leads (II, III, and aVF).

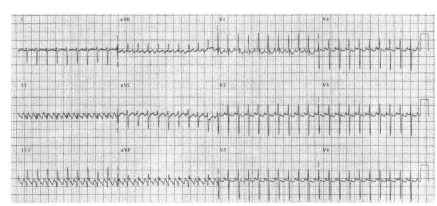

Figure 9.1

Concise Guide to Pediatric Arrhythmias, First Edition. Christopher Wren.
© 2012 John Wiley & Sons, Ltd. Published 2012 by John Wiley & Sons, Ltd.

In Figure 9.2, also from a neonate, AV conduction is slow and variable, producing irregular QRS complexes with aberration in the third and fourth QRS complexes, which follow the shortest RR intervals.

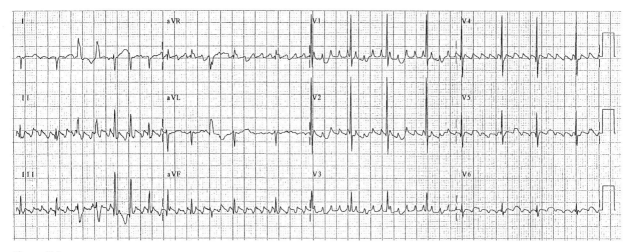

Figure 9.2

Atrial flutter usually has 2:1 AV conduction so the ventricular rate is half the atrial rate and QRS complexes are regular. Sometimes, as in the example in Figure 9.3 from a 10-year-old boy with mitral regurgitation, flutter waves cannot be seen. The diagnosis is suspected from the ventricular rate and confirmed by adenosine administration (see Chapter 6) which increases the AV block to unmask the flutter waves (red arrow on the rhythm strip in Figure 9.4).

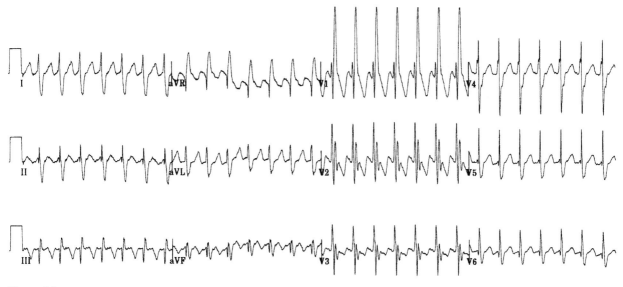

Figure 9.3

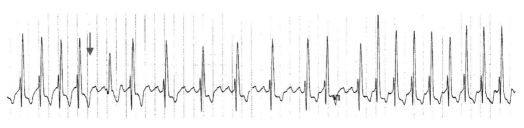

Figure 9.4

Less commonly there is 1:1 AV conduction. This usually occurs when the atrial rate is slowed by drugs or atrial disease. The ECG in Figure 9.5 was recorded immediately after birth from a neonate treated *in utero* with maternal flecainide, which widened the QRS and slowed the flutter rate to about 300/min to allow 1:1 conduction. The ECG in Figure 9.6 is from a young adult late after repair of tetralogy of Fallot. The diagnosis of atrial flutter with 1:1 conduction was confirmed by adenosine administration.

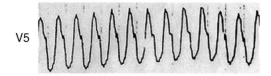

Figure 9.5

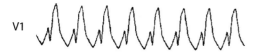

Figure 9.6

Treatment

The first aim of treatment is restoration of sinus rhythm, which is achieved in neonates by transesophageal overdrive pacing or synchronized low-energy DC cardioversion using around 0.5–1 J/kg. In older children with impaired cardiac function or atrial distension, overdrive pacing is less successful and cardioversion is often needed. Recurrence of atrial flutter in neonates is rare and prophylactic medication is not required. In older children attention will be paid to the underlying haemodynamic abnormality, and options for management include drugs, cardiac surgery with or without direct antiarrhythmic surgery, and catheter ablation.

Key references

Campbell RWF. Pharmacologic therapy of atrial flutter. *J Cardiovasc Electrophysiol* 1996;**7**: 1008–12.

Casey FA, McCrindle BW, Hamilton RM, et al. Neonatal atrial flutter: significant early morbidity and excellent long-term prognosis. *Am Heart J* 1997;**133**:302–6.

Garson A Jr, Bink-Boelkens M, Hesslein PS, et al. Atrial flutter in the young: a collaborative study of 380 cases. *J Am Coll Cardiol* 1985;**6**:871–8.

Lisowski LA, Verheijen PM, Benatar AA, et al. Atrial flutter in the perinatal age group: diagnosis, management and outcome. *J Am Coll Cardiol* 2000;**35**:771–7.

Waldo AL. Treatment of atrial flutter. *Heart* 2000;**84**:227–32.

10 Atrial fibrillation

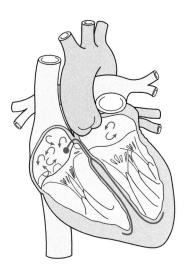

Although common in adults, atrial fibrillation is a rare arrhythmia in childhood. It has mostly been reported in association with rheumatic or congenital heart disease or cardiomyopathy, but it also occurs as an isolated arrhythmia, so-called "lone atrial fibrillation."

There are probably several reasons for the rarity of atrial fibrillation in children. It is caused by multiple small re-entry circuits within the atria. In children the atria are small and may not have sufficient mass to sustain atrial fibrillation. The atria are also less likely to be affected by processes such as chronic fibrosis so the substrate for atrial fibrillation is very unlikely to be present. Lone atrial fibrillation in older children is probably triggered by rapid focal atrial tachycardia in the pulmonary veins or left or right atria, as in adults.

ECG diagnosis

Atrial fibrillation is recognized on the ECG from the absence of P waves and the presence of a chaotic irregular baseline. Atrioventricular (AV) conduction is erratic, producing irregularly irregular QRS complexes. The ventricular rate is usually significantly higher than normal but depends on the characteristics of the AV node and will be lower in the presence of antiarrhythmic drugs.

The example in Figure 10.1 shows atrial fibrillation in a 14-year-old boy. Chaotically irregular atrial activity is well seen, especially in the V1 rhythm strip. The QRS complexes are rapid and irregularly irregular. A few QRS complexes – those following short RR intervals that are preceded by longer RR intervals – are conducted with left bundle branch block (LBBB) aberration, the so-called Ashman phenomenon. The wide QRS complexes should not be mistaken for ventricular premature beats. This was his first episode of atrial fibrillation with no immediately obvious cause. It reverted to sinus rhythm spontaneously and the ECG was then normal. However, ambulatory monitoring revealed ventricular pre-excitation at low heart rates, confirming underlying Wolff–Parkinson–White syndrome. Catheter ablation was successful and there was no recurrence of atrial fibrillation. Atrial fibrillation with

Concise Guide to Pediatric Arrhythmias, First Edition. Christopher Wren.
© 2012 John Wiley & Sons, Ltd. Published 2012 by John Wiley & Sons, Ltd.

pre-excitation is a rare arrhythmia in children with Wolff–Parkinson–White syndrome (see Chapter 13).

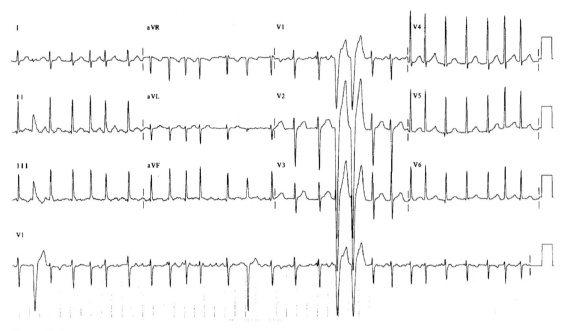

Figure 10.1

Atrial fibrillation is a fairly common early postoperative arrhythmia in young adults who have undergone cardiac surgery (see Chapter 31). The example in Figure 10.2 shows an irregular tachycardia in a 40-year-old woman 2 days after an aortic root replacement. The ECG also shows LBBB.

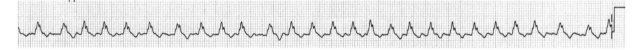

Figure 10.2

Figure 10.3 shows another example of atrial fibrillation in a 15-year-old boy. QRS complexes are irregularly irregular and low amplitude atrial electrical activity is clearly seen in the longer RR intervals. No obvious cause was found, although the arrhythmia may have been related to marked dilation at the connection of the right pulmonary veins to the left atrium identified, on magnetic resonance imaging (MRI) and transesophageal echocardiography.

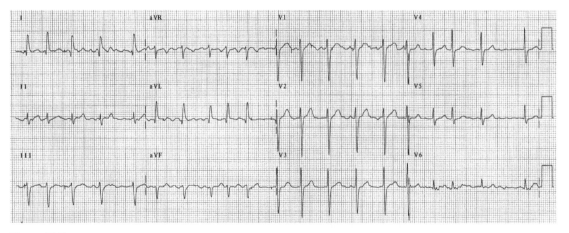

Figure 10.3

Atrial fibrillation is occasionally produced by adenosine injection, as in Figure 10.4. Here adenosine was given in sinus rhythm in an attempt to unmask latent ventricular pre-excitation. In this situation atrial fibrillation is transient and self-correcting.

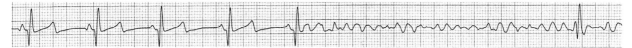

Figure 10.4

Treatment

In adults there are three main strategies for treatment of atrial fibrillation – termination of atrial fibrillation, prevention of recurrence, and ventricular rate control in atrial fibrillation. As atrial fibrillation is so rare in childhood, there is little reported experience of treatment and the management plan will need to be tailored to the individual. In principle, the aim will be to restore sinus rhythm and to look for underlying causes that may be amenable to treatment.

A new episode of atrial fibrillation may resolve spontaneously within a few hours. If it does not, synchronized DC cardioversion will usually restore sinus rhythm. Chemical cardioversion with flecainide or propafenone has some success in adults, with amiodarone reserved for those with poor ventricular function.

Chronic ventricular rate control is probably the least desirable strategy for management of atrial fibrillation in children. The most commonly used agents in adults are calcium channel blockers, β-blockers, digoxin, and amiodarone.

Isolated recurrent or persistent atrial fibrillation in adults is often treated by catheter ablation and this technique may be appropriate for occasional older children if no underlying cause can be identified.

Key references

Blaauw Y, Van Gelder IC, Crijns HJ. Treatment of atrial fibrillation. *Heart* 2002;**88**:432–7.

Fuster V, Rydén LE, Cannom DS, et al. ACC/AHA/ESC 2006 Guidelines for the management of patients with atrial fibrillation: a report of the American College of Cardiology/American Heart Association Task Force on practice guidelines and the European Society of Cardiology Committee for Practice Guidelines (Writing Committee to Revise the 2001 Guidelines for the management of patients with atrial fibrillation). *J Am Coll Cardiol* 2006;**48**:e149–246.

Gow RM. Atrial fibrillation and flutter in children and in young adults with congenital heart disease. *Can J Cardiol* 1996;**12**(suppl A):45A–8A.

Luedtke SA, Kuhn RJ, McCaffrey FM. Pharmacologic management of supraventricular tachycardias in children. Part 2: Atrial flutter, atrial fibrillation, and junctional and atrial ectopic tachycardia. *Ann Pharmacother* 1997;**31**:1347–59.

Markides V, Schilling RJ. Atrial fibrillation: classification, pathophysiology, mechanisms and drug treatment. *Heart* 2003;**89**:939–43.

Nanthakumar K, Lau YR, Plumb VJ, et al. Electrophysiological findings in adolescents with atrial fibrillation who have structurally normal hearts. *Circulation* 2004;**110**:117–23.

Radford DJ, Izukawa T. Atrial fibrillation in children. *Pediatrics* 1977;**59**:250–6.

Rho RW. The management of atrial fibrillation after cardiac surgery. *Heart* 2009;**95**:422–9.

Strieper MJ, Frias, P, Fischbach P, et al. Catheter ablation of primary supraventricular tachycardia substrate presenting as atrial fibrillation in adolescents. *Congen Heart Dis* 2010;**5**:465–9.

11   Atrial premature beats

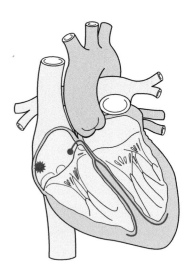

Atrial premature beats, sometimes also known as premature atrial contractions or complexes, are common findings at all ages in infants and children but they rarely cause symptoms. They are usually of no clinical significance and do not require treatment. They often occur too early to be conducted to the ventricles because the atrioventricular (AV) node is still refractory from the previous sinus beat, so there is an apparently "dropped beat" that may be mistaken for AV block.

Atrial premature beats are most often seen in newborn babies and they probably occur even more frequently in fetal life. Although some episodes of common re-entry tachycardias are initiated by atrial premature beats, infants or children who are noted to have frequent atrial premature beats only rarely develop significant arrhythmias.

The premature beat produces a P wave that occurs earlier than expected (red arrow in Figure 11.1), and has a different shape from sinus P waves (this is not always apparent on a single lead recording). Premature P waves are usually superimposed on the previous T wave and can be difficult to identify. If the P wave reaches the AV node before the node has repolarized, conduction will be blocked, as is the case here.

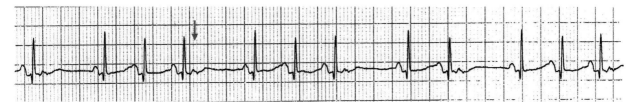

Figure 11.1

Some atrial premature beats may be conducted to the ventricles and others blocked, depending on the degree of prematurity. In the recording in Figure 11.2 some atrial premature beats (black arrows) are conducted with a minor change in QRS morphology. Others (red arrows) are not conducted because they reach the AV node very slightly earlier. The mixture of conducted and non-conducted P waves

Concise Guide to Pediatric Arrhythmias, First Edition. Christopher Wren.
© 2012 John Wiley & Sons, Ltd. Published 2012 by John Wiley & Sons, Ltd.

makes the latter easier to identify. Later conducted atrial premature beats will usually have a normal QRS whereas earlier conducted beats are more likely to produce a partial or complete bundle branch block pattern in the QRS (functional aberration), not to be confused with ventricular premature beats (see Chapter 23).

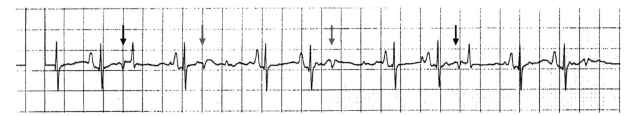

Figure 11.2

In the example in Figure 11.3, from a neonate, every other P wave is premature and is not conducted (red arrows). This rhythm, known as non-conducted atrial bigeminy, should be distinguished from 2:1 AV block (see Chapter 28) by noting the early occurrence and different shape of the premature P waves. It should also not be confused with notched P waves which are common in leads V2 and V3 in older children (see Chapter 4).

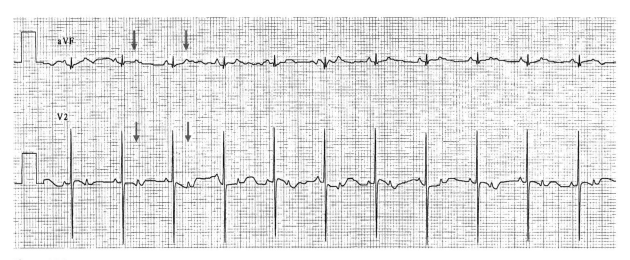

Figure 11.3

Atrial premature beats may occur sporadically or in patterns. If they occur after three sinus beats, as in Figure 11.4, this is known as quadrigeminy. In this example none of the premature beats is conducted.

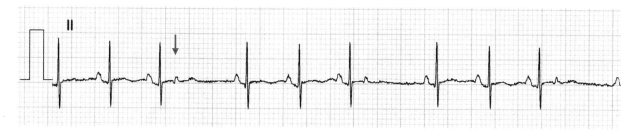

Figure 11.4

If atrial premature beats occur after two sinus beats the pattern is known as trigeminy, as shown in Figure 11.5.

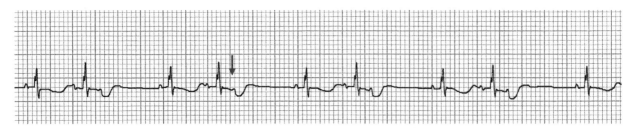

Figure 11.5

In the example in Figure 11.6, from a preterm neonate, all the atrial premature beats are conducted (red arrows) and are followed by a normal QRS. In an older child this pattern might need to be distinguished from respiratory sinus arrhythmia (see Chapter 4).

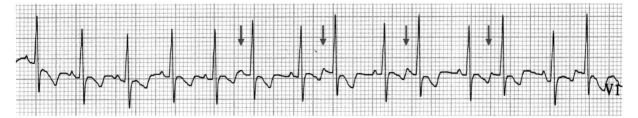

Figure 11.6

In the ECG in Figure 11.7 atrial premature beats are non-conducted (red arrow), conducted with bundle branch block aberration (first black arrow), or conducted with a more or less normal QRS (second black arrow), all depending on very minor changes in the degree of prematurity.

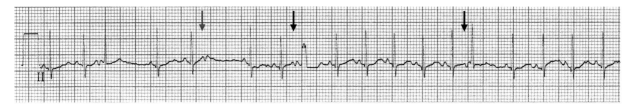

Figure 11.7

Atrial premature beats are common after cardiac surgery but rarely cause significant haemodynamic disturbance. The example in Figure 11.8 shows both conducted (black arrows) and non-conducted (red arrows) atrial premature beats producing alternating bradycardia and tachycardia.

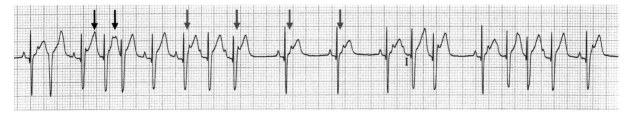

Figure 11.8

Key references

Dickinson DF. The normal ECG in childhood and adolescence. *Heart* 2005;**91**:1626–30.

12 Atrioventricular re-entry tachycardia

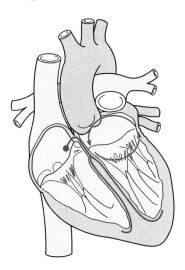

Orthodromic atrioventricular re-entry tachycardia (AVRT) is the most common type of tachycardia found in children at all ages and by far the most common in infancy. (Orthodromic means that the atrioventricular [AV] re-entry circuit runs forward over the AV node.) The substrate for the tachycardia is a small accessory muscular AV connection that connects atrial myocardium to adjacent ventricular myocardium. The re-entry circuit comprises the AV node, ventricle, accessory connection or pathway, and atrium. Accessory pathways can be situated anywhere around the AV junction but the most common position is on the left side of the heart, in the lateral commissure of the mitral valve. Most accessory pathways conduct only retrogradely and so show a normal QRS in both sinus rhythm and tachycardia. A significant minority is capable of anterograde conduction and so will show ventricular pre-excitation in sinus rhythm (see Chapter 13).

ECG diagnosis

The ECG diagnosis of AVRT is usually fairly straightforward. The QRS is usually normal but may show a bundle branch block pattern due to rate-related aberration (see Chapter 5). The rate depends on the age of the child – it is often around 300/min in early infancy, around 250/min in early childhood, and around 200/min in the teenage years. The tachycardia rate gets lower with age – the circuit gets longer as the heart grows, so the cycle length increases. The rate is usually fairly similar in different episodes of tachycardia in the same child. In the example in Figure 12.1, from a neonate, the rate is around 290/min and the QRS is normal. A P wave is clearly seen in lead V1 (labeled C1 on this recording) as shown by the red arrow.

Concise Guide to Pediatric Arrhythmias, First Edition. Christopher Wren.
© 2012 John Wiley & Sons, Ltd. Published 2012 by John Wiley & Sons, Ltd.

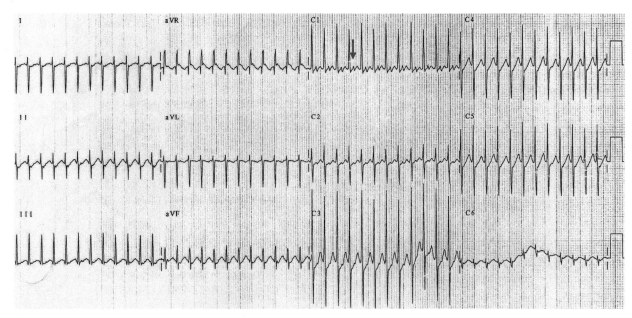

Figure 12.1

If we look more closely at lead V1 in the same ECG (Figure 12.2), the P wave is clearly seen in a position closer to the previous than the following QRS, in the ST segment, i.e. this is a short RP tachycardia (see Chapter 5). P waves in AVRT are usually easiest to see in V1 but may be better seen in other leads so it is important to record a 12-lead ECG.

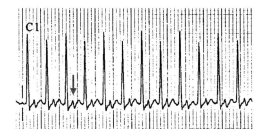

Figure 12.2

P waves are not always easy to see but are usually visible if you look carefully. As mentioned, lead V1 is often the best but P waves may also be seen soon after the QRS in leads II and III or other leads. In Figure 12.3, the P wave in lead III is superimposed on the ST segment (red arrow).

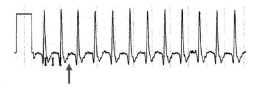

Figure 12.3

Figure 12.4 shows another example of neonatal AVRT. The rate is >300/min and the QRS is very narrow at around 40 ms. P waves are most easily identified in lead

III (black arrow) and in lead (red arrow).

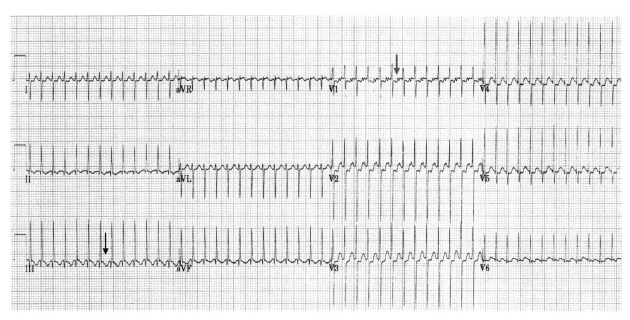

Figure 12.4

The infant in Figure 12.4 was treated with adenosine to stop the tachycardia and Figure 12.5 shows the importance of recording a rhythm strip while doing so. Adenosine produced AV block: tachycardia ends with a non-conducted P wave (first black arrow); the first sinus beat then shows subtle evidence of ventricular pre-excitation (red arrow). The next three QRS complexes are junctional in origin and closely followed by inverted P waves, which are retrogradely conducted over the accessory pathway and have the same morphology as in tachycardia (second black arrow). Sinus rhythm resumes once the adenosine has worn off and the last five sinus beats again show subtle pre-excitation. All these findings are confirmation of the presence of an accessory pathway.

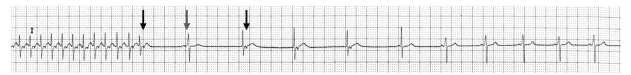

Figure 12.5

AVRT in infants is usually sustained and requires treatment. In older children it is often paroxysmal and self-terminating and may be difficult to document. Holter monitoring is unlikely to be helpful unless the episodes are very frequent but an event recorder can be very useful. Figure 12.6 shows a recording from a 10-year-old boy with palpitations. The arrhythmia is documented but the mechanism cannot be confirmed on this evidence. The differential diagnosis is mainly between AVRT and AV nodal re-entry (see Chapter 16). The presence or absence of ST depression can help in interpretation on the 12-lead ECG recording – the former is more likely in AVRT whereas the latter favors AV nodal re-entry. The timing of the P waves is also helpful (see Chapter 5). The diagnosis of AVRT was proved in this boy at an electrophysiology study before catheter ablation.

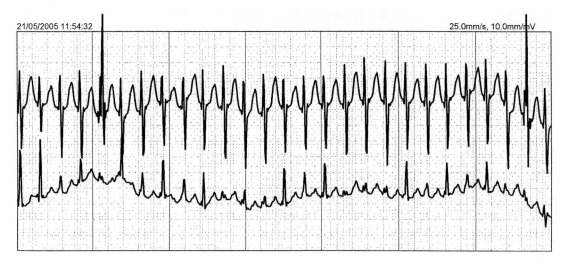

21/05/2005 11:54:32   25.0mm/s, 10.0mm/mV

Figure 12.6

The QRS is usually normal in AVRT, but it is common to see transient rate-related left or right bundle branch block for a few beats at the onset of tachycardia, as shown in Figure 12.7.

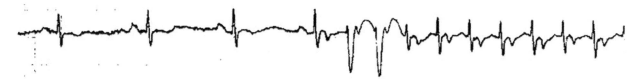

Figure 12.7

AVRT may also occur in infants or children with a sustained bundle branch block pattern – either pre-existing or rate-related (see Chapter 5). Figure 12.8 shows a 12-lead ECG from a neonate. Although sustained left bundle branch block in tachycardia is very unusual in AVRT at this age, AVRT is still the most likely diagnosis. The differential diagnosis includes right ventricular tachycardia, atriofascicular re-entry (see Chapter 15), and antidromic re-entry (see Chapter 13). The first is rare at this age and the last two occur only in older children.

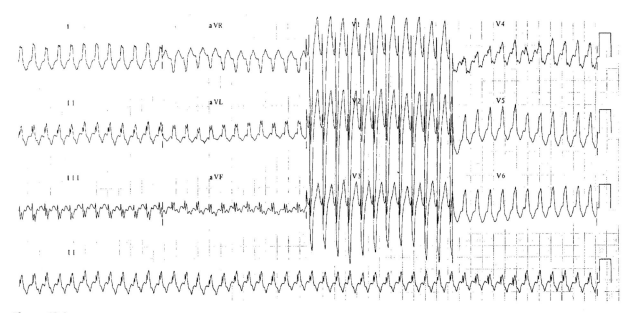

Figure 12.8

Sustained bundle branch block also occurs in older children. Figure 12.9 shows an ECG from an 8-year-old boy with AVRT. The QRS shows typical right bundle branch block morphology. The differential diagnosis here includes other types of SVT with right bundle branch block, antidromic re-entry, and left ventricular tachycardia (see Chapter 5). If ECG recordings of other episodes of tachycardia in the same child show normal QRS complexes the last of these is excluded as a possibility.

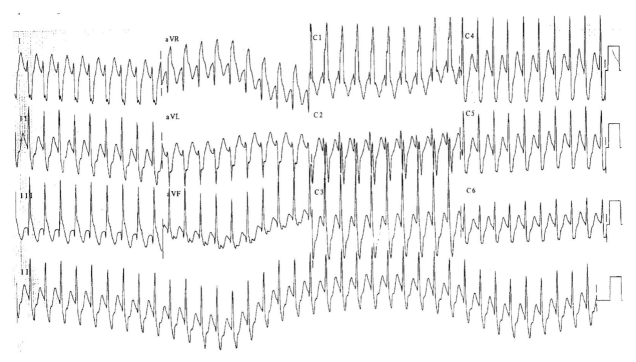

Figure 12.9

Occasionally the ECG will show transient bundle branch block associated with a change in ventricular rate. Figure 12.10 shows five beats with left bundle branch block just after the start of tachycardia. As the block resolves the tachycardia cycle length shortens (i.e. the rate increases). This is compelling evidence for an accessory pathway on the same side as the bundle branch block (contralateral bundle branch block does not affect the rate).

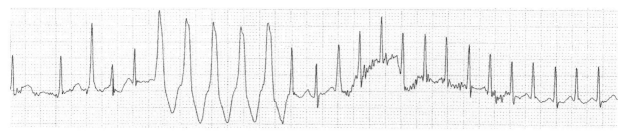

Figure 12.10

Differential diagnosis

The diagnosis in infancy is usually clear with a presentation with heart failure and a rate of 270/min or more (occasionally slightly slower in preterm infants). AVRT in infancy should be distinguished from permanent junctional re-entry tachycardia by examining the ECG (see Chapter 5) and from atrial tachycardia, which will show some degree of AV block, with or without adenosine (see Chapter 6). AVRT in older children should be distinguished from AV nodal re-entry (see Chapter 16). The distinction is mainly important if one is considering catheter ablation because both respond acutely to adenosine.

Treatment of AVRT

In infancy

The immediate aim of treatment of sustained AVRT is the restoration of sinus rhythm. In the newborn baby this is best achieved with intravenous adenosine in a dose of 150–250 μg/kg or occasionally more (see Chapters 6 and 37). Facial application of ice-cold water or an ice pack is effective, and was more often used in the past, but it is suitable only for very young infants. Eyeball pressure should not be used for fear of causing damage to the eyes. Verapamil should not be used in infancy.

In the short term the risk of recurrence of AVRT in infants is fairly high, so prophylactic antiarrhythmic medication should be given. Infants were most often treated with either digoxin or a β-blocker in the past, although the efficacy of these drugs is probably not high. All published reports of drug treatment of tachycardia in infancy are retrospective uncontrolled observational studies, so the effect of treatment is difficult to assess. Newer drugs such as flecainide and amiodarone are probably significantly more effective but should be prescribed only by those familiar with their use. Prophylactic medication is usually given for 6–12 months and after that time most infants will have no further recurrence. Those who do can be managed as below. Persistence of a Wolff–Parkinson–White pattern on the ECG gives a significantly higher chance of recurrence of tachycardia.

In childhood

Termination of tachycardia in older children can sometimes be achieved by vagal maneuvers, such as a Valsalva maneuver or carotid massage. Otherwise AVRT will almost always respond to intravenous adenosine in a dose of 100–250 μg/kg or verapamil 100–300 μg/kg.

If tachycardia develops or continues after the age of 5 years, long-term spontaneous resolution is very unlikely. AVRT is not an intrinsically dangerous arrhythmia so further management will depend on the frequency, severity, and duration of attacks. If they are infrequent, short lasting, and easily controlled, or self-terminating no treatment will be required. Otherwise the choice is between regular antiarrhythmic medication (generally not a very satisfactory long-term solution) and catheter ablation (see Chapter 39). AVRT in a child with pre-excitation on the ECG in sinus rhythm is usually seen as a strong indication for an electrophysiology study with a view to catheter ablation.

Key references

Delacretaz E. Supraventricular tachycardia. *N Engl J Med* 2006;**354**:1039–51.

Gilljam T, Jaeggi E, Gow RM. Neonatal supraventricular tachycardia: outcomes over a 27-year period at a single institution. *Acta Paediatr* 2008;**97**:1035–9.

Jaeggi ET, Gilljam T, Bauersfeld U, et al. Electrocardiographic differentiation of typical atrioventricular node reentrant tachycardia from atrioventricular reciprocating tachycardia mediated by concealed accessory pathway in children. *Am J Cardiol* 2003;**91**:1084–9.

Tortoriello T, Snyder C, O'Brian Smith E, et al. Frequency of recurrence among infants with supraventricular tachycardia and comparison of recurrence rates among those with and without preexcitation and among those with and without response to digoxin and/or propranolol therapy. *Am J Cardiol* 2003;**92**:1045–9.

Weindling SN, Saul JP, Walsh EP. Efficacy and risks of medical therapy for supraventricular tachycardia in neonates and infants. *An Heart J* 1996;**131**:66–72.

Wong KK, Potts JE, Etheridge SP, et al. Medications used to manage supraventricular tachycardia in the infant. A North American survey. *Pediatr Cardiol* 2006;**27**:199–203.

13   Wolff–Parkinson–White syndrome

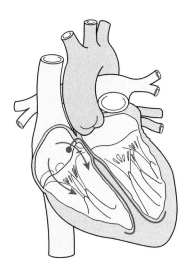

Wolff–Parkinson–White (WPW) syndrome describes the combination of ventricular pre-excitation in sinus rhythm with paroxysmal tachycardia. Isolated pre-excitation in the absence of any arrhythmia is perhaps better described as an ECG showing the WPW pattern. The substrate for pre-excitation is an accessory muscular atrioventricular (AV) connection (accessory pathway). Accessory pathways are short muscular connections between the atrial myocardium and the adjacent ventricular myocardium. They are usually very small and can occur almost anywhere around the AV junction. Pathways on the left side are more common but they also occur in the middle of the heart or on the right. Most are single but some patients have more than one, more often on the right.

The most common arrhythmia seen in WPW syndrome is orthodromic AV re-entry tachycardia (see Chapter 12), but antidromic re-entry and atrial fibrillation also occur (see below).

Apart from a few rare arrhythmias discussed below, pre-excitation is evident only in sinus rhythm. It is caused by simultaneous AV conduction over the normal conduction axis and the accessory pathway, with fusion of the two waves of activation of the ventricles. Pre-excitation is usually persistent but may be intermittent or latent (i.e. only produced when the AV node is suppressed).

ECG diagnosis

The hallmark of pre-excitation is a short PR interval and a widened QRS with slow early activation – the delta wave (usually a slurred upstroke if the QRS is positive). In Figure 13.1 AV re-entry tachycardia is terminated with verapamil, a drug that affects the AV node but not the accessory pathway. In tachycardia the QRS is normal, because all ventricular activation occurs via the His bundle, whereas retrograde conduction from the ventricle to the atrium completes the re-entry circuit. When tachycardia breaks, sinus rhythm is restored, and pre-excitation becomes obvious – compare the PR interval and QRS appearance in normally conducted (black arrow) and pre-excited (red arrow) beats.

Concise Guide to Pediatric Arrhythmias, First Edition. Christopher Wren.
© 2012 John Wiley & Sons, Ltd. Published 2012 by John Wiley & Sons, Ltd.

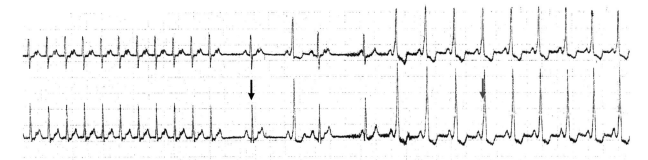

Figure 13.1

The degree of pre-excitation varies between patients and may be obvious or subtle. A left-sided pathway is farther away from the sinus node than one on the right and the atrial impulse takes longer to reach the left atrium. Pre-excitation may be less easy to see with a left-sided pathway (Figure 13.2) and is often more marked (with a more prominent delta wave) in a right-sided pathway (Figure 13.3).

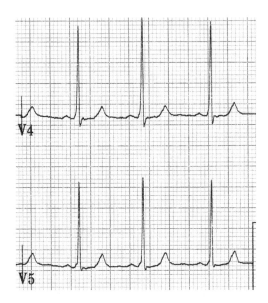

Figure 13.2

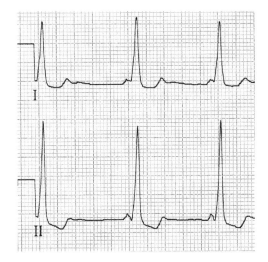

Figure 13.3

The pattern of ventricular pre-excitation depends on the position of the accessory pathway. Figure 13.4 shows a right-sided pathway. Early activation of the right ventricle mimics late activation of the left ventricle and so produces a pattern resembling left bundle branch block (for a more detailed explanation see Chapter 5).

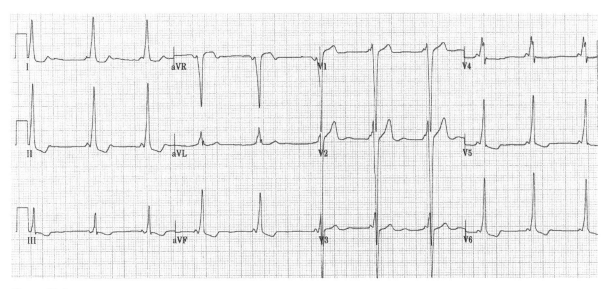

Figure 13.4

In Figure 13.5 the pathway is on the left with dominant R waves in V1–3. Pre-excitation is less obvious – a common feature of left-sided pathways because it takes longer for atrial activation to reach the pathway than the AV node.

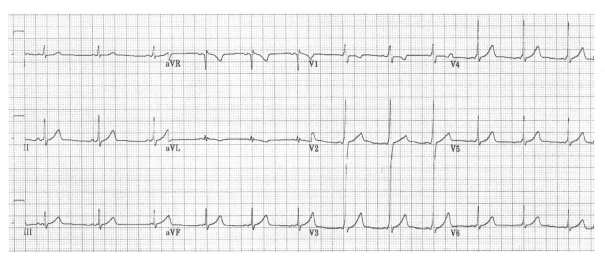

Figure 13.5

In Figure 13.6 the accessory pathway is close to the normal conduction axis in a so-called right midseptal or right anteroseptal position – a potential hazard if radiofrequency ablation is being considered. There are several published algorithms for predicting accessory pathway position from the 12-lead ECG, although none of them is very accurate.

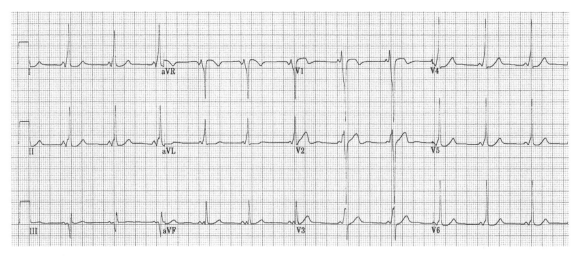

Figure 13.6

The most common arrhythmia by far in WPW syndrome is *orthodromic* AV re-entry tachycardia (see Chapter 12). The QRS complex in tachycardia is usually normal, although it may show transient or sustained bundle branch block, as discussed in Chapter 5. Ventricular pre-excitation will become manifest only once sinus rhythm is restored. Acute management of orthodromic AV re-entry involves termination of tachycardia with vagal maneuvers or adenosine.

Less commonly patients with WPW syndrome will develop *antidromic* AV re-entry tachycardia. This occurs when there is more than one accessory pathway and is more common with right-sided pathways. Anterograde AV conduction occurs over the accessory pathway whereas retrograde conduction is via the His bundle or a second pathway. Antidromic AV re-entry tachycardia is rarely if ever seen in infancy and usually occurs only in older children.

Antidromic AV re-entry tachycardia is regular and the QRS is maximally pre-excited, in effect showing a very prominent delta wave. P waves are usually very difficult to see. With a right-sided pathway the QRS resembles left bundle branch block with a slurred upstroke, as shown in Figure 13.7. Antidromic AV re-entry tachycardia will stop with adenosine if retrograde conduction is over the AV node, but rarely will require intravenous flecainide or cardioversion if two accessory pathways are involved in the circuit.

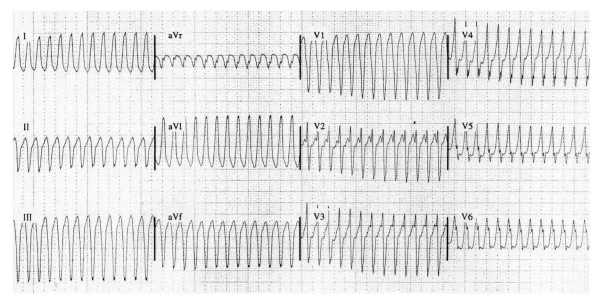

Figure 13.7

Less common is antidromic AV re-entry with a left-sided pathway. We can predict that this will show a QRS similar to a right bundle branch block pattern with a slurred onset, as shown in Figure 13.8.

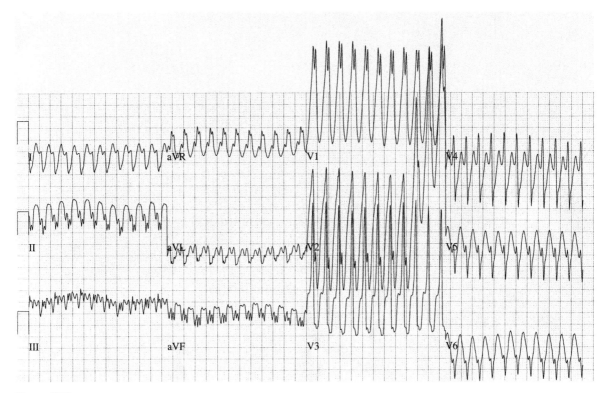

Figure 13.8

One of the least common, but potentially most dangerous, tachycardias in WPW syndromes is atrial fibrillation (AF). This is rare in pediatric practice but presents a risk of syncope or sudden death in a patient with an accessory pathway that has a short refractory period. In pre-excited AF the QRS is maximally pre-excited as seen earlier (because AV conduction is over the pathway) but the rhythm is irregularly irregular, as shown in Figure 13.9.

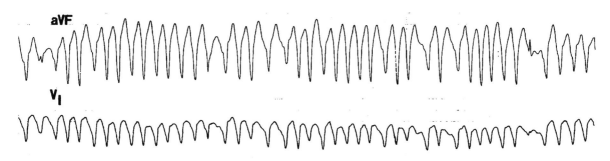

Figure 13.9

AF probably develops most often as a spontaneous degeneration from orthodromic AV re-entry tachycardia, as shown in Figure 13.10.

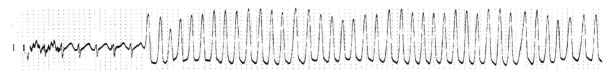

Figure 13.10

If the ventricular rate is high the irregularity can be difficult to make out. Atrial fibrillation with pre-excitation is often mistaken for ventricular tachycardia but, as the management of both involves urgent synchronized DC cardioversion, this is not a major problem. Pre-excitation will be evident on the ECG once cardioversion has restored sinus rhythm. Do not make the correct diagnosis and then give digoxin for the AF because this may well precipitate ventricular fibrillation.

Treatment

Longer-term management of WPW syndrome depends on the arrhythmia, the clinical situation, and the age of the child. AV re-entry tachycardia is treated in the same way whether or not pre-excitation is present. Antiarrhythmic drugs are used in infancy – most commonly a β-blocker, flecainide, or amiodarone (the last two probably being more effective). The choice of drug depends on clinician preference and experience, and on the clinical condition on presentation. It was said in the past that digoxin presented some theoretical risk in pre-excitation, but there is probably no indication for its use in any case because it has little antiarrhythmic effect in this situation.

In older children the treatment of choice is catheter ablation (see Chapter 39). Success rates are high and the need for long-term antiarrhythmic drugs is avoided. The occurrence of antidromic AV re-entry tachycardia or pre-excited AF is probably an absolute indication for invasive investigation and ablation.

There is much debate about whether catheter ablation is indicated for ventricular pre-excitation in the absence of symptoms (so-called asymptomatic WPW syndrome). There is a fine balance between the small risk of the procedure and the very small risk of adverse events if left untreated. The decision will come down to individual choice after discussion with parents and children. "Risk stratification," based on non-invasive or invasive investigation, is of little or no benefit and there is probably no indication for pathway analysis by electrophysiology study.

Key references

Campbell RM, Strieper MJ, Frias PA, et al. Survey of current practice of pediatric electrophysiologists for asymptomatic Wolff–Parkinson–White syndrome. *Pediatrics* 2003;**111**:e245–7.

Dubin AM, Collins KK, Chiesa N, et al. Use of electrophysiologic testing to assess risk in children with Wolff–Parkinson–White syndrome. *Cardiol Young* 2002;**12**:248–52.

Fox DJ, Klein GJ, Skanes AC, et al. How to identify the location of an accessory pathway by the 12-lead ECG. *Heart Rhythm* 2008;**5**:1763–6.

Moss AJ. History of Wolff–Parkinson–White syndrome: introductory note to a classic article by Louis Wolff, M.D., John Parkinson, M.D., and Paul D. White, M.D. *Ann Noninvasive Electrocardiol* 2006;**11**:338–9.

Munger TM, Packer DL, Hammill SC, et al. A population study of the natural history of Wolff–Parkinson–White syndrome in Olmsted County, Minnesota, 1953-1989. *Circulation* 1993;**87**:866–73.

Wellens HJ, Rodriguez LM, Timmermans C, et al. The asymptomatic patient with the Wolff-Parkinson-White electrocardiogram. *Pacing Clin Electrophysiol* 1997;**20**:2082–6.

14 Permanent junctional reciprocating tachycardia

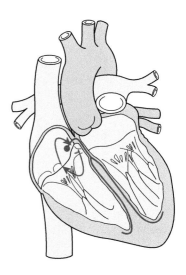

Permanent junctional reciprocating tachycardia (PJRT) was first described by Philippe Coumel in Paris. It is a rare type of orthodromic atrioventricular (AV) re-entry tachycardia, with anterograde conduction through the AV node and retrograde conduction through a concealed accessory pathway (usually just anterior to the mouth of the coronary sinus), which has very slow retrograde conduction. This characteristic means that it is very easy for the tachycardia to start and it is often incessant. It may present at any age in childhood, or even in fetal life, but most cases present in infancy. It may be an incidental finding but often presents with an apparent dilated cardiomyopathy that results from incessant tachycardia. Tachycardia rates vary considerably in different patients, from 300/min in neonates to 150/min or less in asymptomatic children. PJRT is rarely associated with structural heart disease.

ECG diagnosis

The mechanism of the tachycardia accounts for the ECG appearances. The QRS is normal for age and P waves are clearly seen with a 1:1 AV relationship. The P wave is much closer to the following QRS so this is a type of long RP tachycardia. The P waves are characteristically deeply inverted in leads II, III, and aVF, as shown in Figure 14.1 (black arrows), because the atria are activated first in the low right atrium. This ECG is from a neonate and the rate is around 240/min.

Concise Guide to Pediatric Arrhythmias, First Edition. Christopher Wren.
© 2012 John Wiley & Sons, Ltd. Published 2012 by John Wiley & Sons, Ltd.

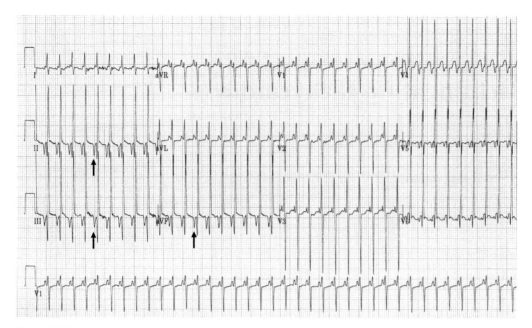

Figure 14.1

In the example in Figure 14.2, the inverted P waves (red arrows) overlap the T waves, which can make it more difficult to be sure of the diagnosis. The differential diagnosis of a long RP tachycardia includes sinus tachycardia and focal atrial tachycardia (see Chapter 5). Sinus tachycardia will obviously have a P wave with a normal axis. The shape of the P wave in atrial tachycardia varies but rarely mimics that shown here in PJRT.

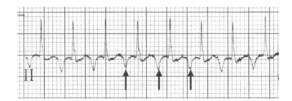

Figure 14.2

Figure 14.3 is another example from a slightly older child to show the consistency of the ECG appearances.

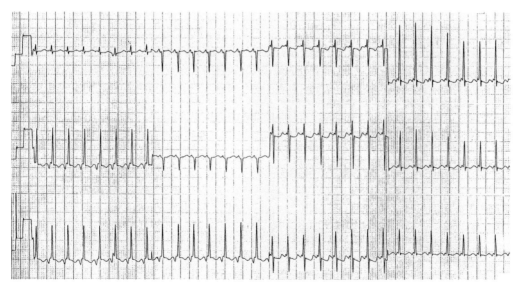

Figure 14.3

Adenosine will usually help if there is any doubt about the diagnosis. PJRT is a re-entry tachycardia with the AV node as part of the re-entry circuit, so adenosine will terminate tachycardia. Tachycardia usually slows before termination, and usually stops with block in the retrograde pathway (identified by termination with a QRS with no following P wave), as shown in Figure 14.4. However, PJRT will often restart as soon as the adenosine has worn off, within a few seconds.

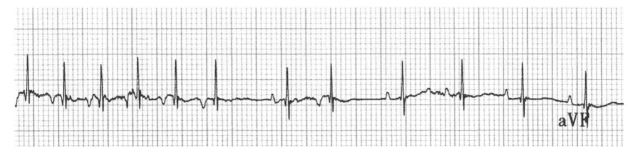

Figure 14.4

Treatment

Management is influenced by the age and clinical condition of the child at presentation. Antiarrhythmic drug treatment is almost always used in infancy. If the function of the left ventricle is significantly impaired, the drug of choice is probably amiodarone. If ventricular function is satisfactory, flecainide or propafenone will usually prove effective. Success is also reported with oral verapamil, although β-blockers and digoxin are less effective. The aim of drug treatment is suppression of the PJRT, although intermittent tachycardia at low rates on Holter monitoring is acceptable. Once control or suppression of tachycardia has been achieved the ventricular function will improve and usually return to normal.

Spontaneous resolution of PJRT is uncommon but is reported in up to 20% of cases during follow-up. In most this is a long-term problem and catheter ablation will usually be recommended. The success of the procedure is lower in smaller patients but overall cure rates are high with either radiofrequency or cryoablation.

Key references

Dorostkar PC, Silka MJ, Morady F, et al. Clinical course of persistent junctional reciprocating tachycardia. *J Am Coll Cardiol* 1999;**33**:366–75.

Drago F, Silvetti MS, Mazza A, et al. Permanent junctional reciprocating tachycardia in infants and children: effectiveness of medical and non-medical treatment. *Ital Heart J* 2001;**2**:456–61.

Gaita F, Montefusco A, Riccardi R, et al. Cryoenergy Catheter Ablation: A new technique for treatment of permanent junctional reciprocating tachycardia in children. *J Cardiovasc Electrophysiol* 2004;**15**:263–8.

Lindinger A, Heisel A, Von Bernuth G, et al. Permanent junctional re-entry tachycardia: a multicenter long-term follow-up study in infants, children and young adults. *Eur Heart J* 1998;**19**:936–42.

Vaksmann G, D'Hoinne C, Lucet V, et al. Permanent junctional reciprocating tachycardia in children: a multicentre study on clinical profile and outcome. *Heart* 2006;**92**:101–4.

van Stuijvenberg M, Beaufort-Krol GC, Haaksma J, et al. Pharmacological treatment of young children with permanent junctional reciprocating tachycardia. *Cardiol Young* 2003;**13**:408–12.

15 Atriofascicular re-entry tachycardia

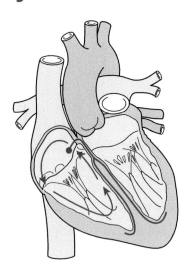

Atriofascicular re-entry is a rare form of supraventricular tachycardia. It was previously erroneously known as "Mahaim tachycardia" because of earlier confusion over the mechanism. It is now known to be an unusual form of antidromic atrioventricular (AV) re-entry. The substrate is an accessory AV connection situated in the right lateral aspect of the tricuspid valve ring. This is thought to be an atriofascicular tract connecting the right atrium to the right bundle branch (the fascicular connection), thus differing from more common accessory AV connections, which are short muscular connections between atrial and ventricular myocardium. The histological evidence for such a pathway is lacking but it would probably be similar to the so-called Kent bundle, which was previously thought (probably wrongly) to be the substrate for the Wolff–Parkinson–White syndrome. It is possible that the substrate of atriofascicular re-entry is anatomically a more common pathway with atypical electrophysiological behavior. The connection exhibits AV node-like properties, with decremental conduction at electrophysiology study and sensitivity to adenosine. Atriofascicular pathways are sometimes associated with Ebstein's malformation of the tricuspid valve and may coexist with typical accessory pathways.

Atriofascicular re-entry tachycardia is a type of antidromic AV re-entry (see Chapter 13). The arrhythmia circuit comprises anterograde conduction over the anomalous connection to the distal right bundle branch and retrograde conduction through the His bundle and AV node to the right atrium. As a result of this the QRS in tachycardia is always abnormal. It shows left bundle branch block morphology because, in effect, the tachycardia pre-excites the right bundle branch.

ECG diagnosis

The ECG in sinus rhythm is normal, with no pre-excitation. The ECG in tachycardia, as mentioned above, shows a left bundle branch block pattern, often with left axis deviation, as shown in Figure 15.1. Unlike pre-excited tachycardia in Wolff–Parkinson–White syndrome, the ECG here shows a rapid onset to the QRS, more like typical left bundle branch block. The rate here is 205/min.

Concise Guide to Pediatric Arrhythmias, First Edition. Christopher Wren.
© 2012 John Wiley & Sons, Ltd. Published 2012 by John Wiley & Sons, Ltd.

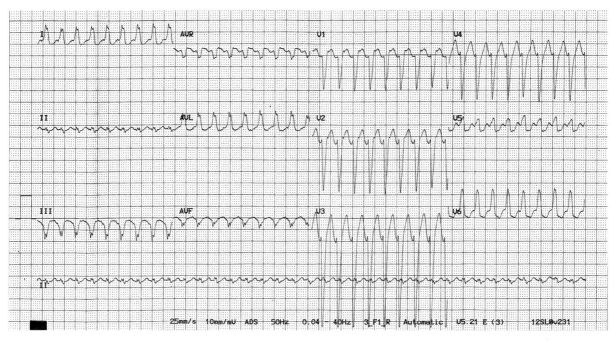

Figure 15.1

The differential diagnosis is with other forms of tachycardia showing left bundle branch block. This includes other forms of supraventricular tachycardia (SVT) with rate-related or pre-existing left bundle branch block, antidromic AV re-entry with a right-sided accessory connection, and ventricular tachycardia originating in the right ventricle, although the last two will have a rather different QRS morphology (see Chapter 5). Faced with a child with this ECG for the first time, it is not possible to distinguish atriofascicular re-entry tachycardia from a more common type of SVT with left bundle branch block aberration. If a subsequent episode of tachycardia shows a normal QRS, the diagnosis cannot be atriofascicular re-entry. If several different episodes all show a left bundle branch block pattern, atriofascicular re-entry becomes more likely.

In the example in Figure 15.2, from a 14-year-old girl, a very similar QRS pattern is observed with a ventricular rate of 170/min. P waves cannot be seen with any certainty. Again there is left axis deviation. Atriofascicular re-entry tachycardia usually occurs in teenagers rather than younger children and is probably more common in girls.

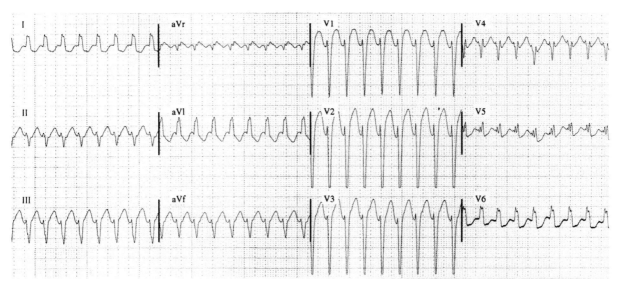

Figure 15.2

Figure 15.3 is from a younger patient – a 9-year-old girl. The rate is higher at 225/min. This time there is an inferior QRS axis.

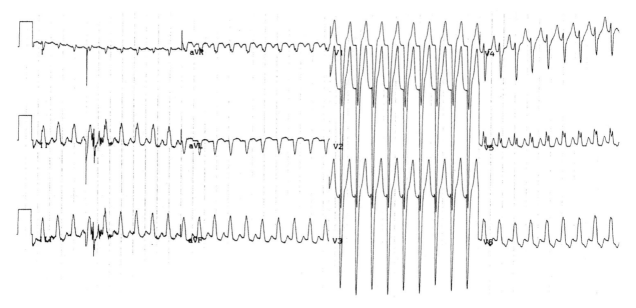

Figure 15.3

Treatment

Atriofascicular re-entry tachycardia responds acutely to adenosine. In the long run it is probably best treated by radiofrequency catheter ablation as the response to prophylactic drug treatment is said to be poor. The abnormal connection is usually localized by recording a sharp local electrogram, similar to a His bundle spike, and the cure rate from ablation is high.

Key references

Aliot E, de Chillou C, Revault d'Allones G, et al. Mahaim tachycardias. *Eur Heart* J 1998; **19**(suppl E): 25–31.

Anderson RH, Ho SY, Gillette PC, et al. Mahaim, Kent and abnormal atrioventricular conduction. *Cardiovasc Res* 1996;**31**:480–91.

Benditt DG, Lü F. Atriofascicular pathways: fuzzy nomenclature or merely wishful thinking? *J Cardiovasc Electrophysiol* 2006;**17**:261–5.

Ellenbogen KA, Vijayaraman P. Mahaim fibers: new electrophysiologic insights into an unusual variant. *J Cardiovasc Electrophysiol* 2005;**16**:135–6.

Klein GJ, Guiraudon G, Guiraudon C, et al. The nodoventricular Mahaim pathway: an endangered concept? *Circulation* 1994;**90**:636–8.

16 Atrioventricular nodal re-entry tachycardia

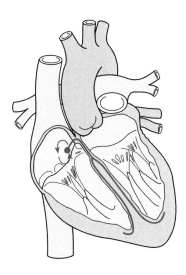

Atrioventricular (AV) nodal re-entry tachycardia (AVNRT), sometimes also known as AV nodal *re-entrant* tachycardia or AV *junctional* re-entry tachycardia, is the second most common type of supraventricular tachycardia in children. It rarely, if ever, occurs in infants and is rare before school age, becoming progressively more common in later childhood.

AV nodal re-entry tachycardia is a typical re-entry arrhythmia. It is paroxysmal and can be stopped and started by pacing. It might be better known as atrionodal re-entry, because the arrhythmia circuit comprises the AV node and adjacent low right atrium. There is no proven anatomical substrate, but it has been suggested recently that the inferior extensions of the AV node may be the anatomical substrate of the "slow pathway."

AV nodal re-entry usually presents with palpitations, sometimes associated with dizziness, breathlessness, or a feeling of fullness in the neck. Episodes of tachycardia may be very frequent, with several in a day. (This frequency would be unusual in AV re-entry with a concealed accessory pathway, which is the main differential diagnosis.)

The ECG in tachycardia almost always shows a normal QRS because sustained rate-related aberration is rare. The QRS complexes are regular and the rate usually between 150 and 250/min. Variations in rate between different episodes of tachycardia are greater than is seen in AV re-entry. Figure 16.1 shows a typical episode from a 15-year-old boy. Note the normal QRS and the initial difficulty in identifying a P wave.

Concise Guide to Pediatric Arrhythmias, First Edition. Christopher Wren.
© 2012 John Wiley & Sons, Ltd. Published 2012 by John Wiley & Sons, Ltd.

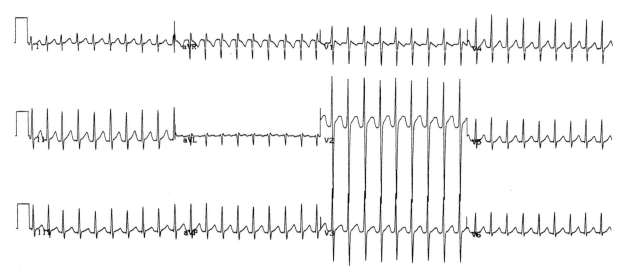

Figure 16.1

Although P waves are not easy to see in AVNRT they are usually visible if one knows where to look. Atrial and ventricular activation are almost simultaneous so the P wave is nearly hidden behind the QRS. It produces a small positive deflection at the end of the QRS in lead V1, which looks a bit like an r′ wave (red arrow). It is helpful to compare with the appearance in the same lead after restoration of sinus rhythm, as shown in Figure 16.2, where the same positive defection is not seen.

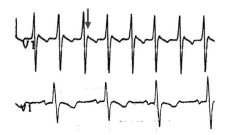

Figure 16.2

Four more examples in Figure 16.3 show how reproducible this appearance is. All recordings show lead V1. Again there is a pseudo r′ in tachycardia (red arrows in upper traces) and this is not present in sinus rhythm (lower traces).

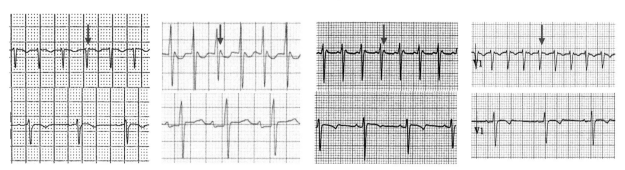

Figure 16.3

Sometimes the RP interval in AVRT is slightly longer than usual, and the ECG may then show pseudo S waves in inferior and lateral leads (black arrows in Figure 16.4). The P wave is also seen as a positive deflection in lead V1 (red arrow) but slightly later than the examples in Figures 16.2 and 16.3. AVNRT was proven at electrophysiology study in this 14-year-old girl. If there is doubt about which is the

P wave it is very helpful to compare with the QRS morphology in sinus rhythm – as shown in Figure 16.5 for this patient.

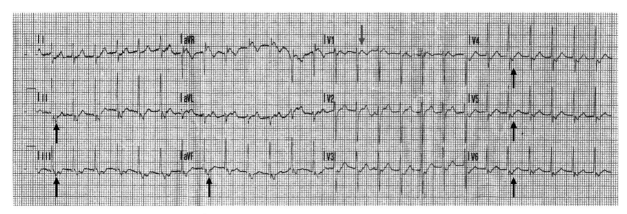

Figure 16.4

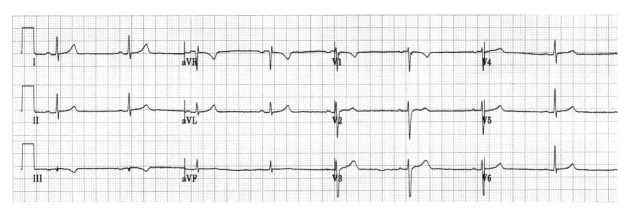

Figure 16.5

Acute treatment of AV nodal re-entry is aimed at restoration of sinus rhythm. Vagal maneuvers are sometimes effective. Otherwise tachycardia can be terminated with intravenous adenosine or verapamil.

The choice of long-term treatment depends on the frequency, severity, and duration of symptoms. A wait-and-see approach is reasonable if episodes of tachycardia are infrequent, short lasting, and self-limiting. Otherwise the choice is prophylactic antiarrhythmic medication or radiofrequency modification of the AV node (see Chapter 39). An oral β-blocker is probably the drug of choice and success may also be obtained with oral verapamil or flecainide.

Although AV nodal re-entry may be suspected from the clinical history and ECG appearances, most often the diagnosis is proven only at an electrophysiology study. This means that in many cases AV re-entry tachycardia remains a possible alternative diagnosis. Many children and their parents will choose invasive investigation that will confirm the diagnosis and also offer the prospect of cure. Radiofrequency modification of the AV node (targeted at the slow pathway along the rim of the tricuspid valve, just anterior to the mouth of the coronary sinus) offers a success rate of >90% with a low risk (<1%) of producing permanent AV block. Cryomodification of the slow pathway is a newer treatment with a reported lower complication rate but also a higher recurrence rate.

Key references

Collins KK, Dubin AM, Chiesa NA, et al. Cryoablation versus radiofrequency ablation for treatment of pediatric atrioventricular nodal reentrant tachycardia: initial experience with 4-mm cryocatheter. *Heart Rhythm* 2006;**3**:571–2.

Drago F, Grutter G, Silvetti MS, et al. Atrioventricular nodal reentrant tachycardia in children. *Pediatr Cardiol* 2006;**27**:454–9.

Jaeggi ET, Gilljam T, Bauersfeld U, et al. Electrocardiographic differentiation of typical atrioventricular node reentrant tachycardia from atrioventricular reciprocating tachycardia mediated by concealed accessory pathway in children. *Am J Cardiol* 2003;**91**:1084–9.

Katritsis DG, Becker A. The atrioventricular nodal reentrant tachycardia circuit: a proposal. *Heart Rhythm* 2007;**4**:1354–60.

Katritsis DG, Camm AJ. Atrioventricular nodal reentrant tachycardia. *Circulation* 2010;**122**:831–40.

Silka MJ, Kron J, Halperin BD, et al. Mechanisms of AV node re-entrant tachycardia in young patients with and without dual AV node physiology. *PACE* 1994;**17**:2129–33.

Junctional ectopic tachycardia

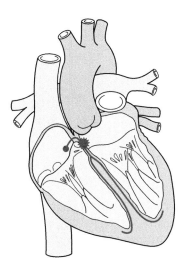

Junctional ectopic tachycardia (JET), sometimes also known as His bundle tachycardia, is a rare arrhythmia most often encountered as an early postoperative complication after open repair of congenital heart malformations (see Chapter 31). However, it may also be seen as a chronic arrhythmia in infants and children in the absence of any structural heart abnormality (and is then known as congenital or idiopathic JET), which sometimes occurs as a familial problem. JET belongs to the uncommon group of tachycardias classified as *ectopic* or *automatic*, in which part of the heart (in this case close to the His bundle) has rapid pacemaker activity. Early postoperative JET is caused by damage to tissues in or around the His bundle from traction, hemorrhage, edema, etc. The cause of congenital JET is unknown. The tachycardia rate in neonates ranges from 150/min to 300/min and postoperatively is usually >170/min.

ECG diagnosis

The ECG shows an unusual pattern with P waves (red arrows) that are slower than, and dissociated from, the QRS complexes, as seen in Figure 17.1. The QRS is usually

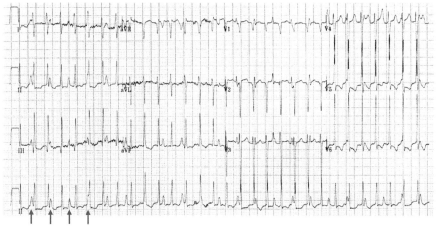

Figure 17.1

Concise Guide to Pediatric Arrhythmias, First Edition. Christopher Wren.
© 2012 John Wiley & Sons, Ltd. Published 2012 by John Wiley & Sons, Ltd.

normal for the child, which obviously means that it may show a right bundle branch block pattern after repair of, for example, tetralogy of Fallot.

In Figure 17.2 the dissociated P waves are clearly seen. The atrial rate (arrows) is around 120/min whereas the ventricular rate is around 190/min.

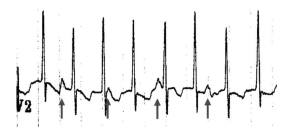

Figure 17.2

The QRS complexes in postoperative JET are usually regular. Sometimes, particularly in congenital JET, they may show occasional irregularity, especially at lower ventricular rates. This is caused by both capture and fusion beats, as is also seen in ventricular tachycardia and discussed in Chapter 18. In Figure 17.3 the P waves (black arrows) are slower than, and dissociated from, the QRS complexes. Occasionally a P wave occurs at a time when it can be conducted to the ventricles, producing an earlier QRS – a capture beat (red arrows).

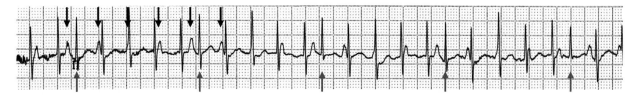

Figure 17.3

Sometimes in postoperative JET there is 1:1 retrograde ventriculoatrial (VA) conduction which makes it difficult to distinguish from other tachycardias with a 1:1 atrioventricular (AV) relationship. However, the response to adenosine will make the diagnosis clear by producing retrograde block, as shown in Figure 17.4. The pattern changes from 1:1 retrograde conduction (with invisible P waves) to show clearly dissociated P waves as indicated by the red arrows.

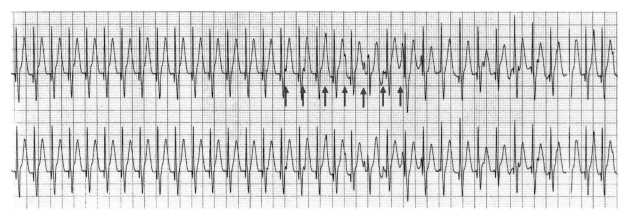

Figure 17.4

JET has true automatic behavior, typically being incessant and unresponsive to overdrive pacing, cardioversion, adenosine, etc. The management plan depends on the clinical situation.

Treatment

Congenital JET may present with heart failure from tachycardia-induced cardiomyopathy, or may be noticed incidentally. It is usually incessant and is treated with a drug that suppresses automaticity, such as flecainide, propafenone, amiodarone. Digoxin, β-blockers, and calcium channel blockers are ineffective. Treatment is continued for several years and the spontaneous tachycardia rate may slow over time, sometimes allowing treatment to be withdrawn. There have been several reports of treatment by radiofrequency ablation or cryoablation, but the risk of AV block is high and the arrhythmia may well resolve over time.

When JET is encountered as an early postoperative arrhythmia, general measures include reduction of dose or withdrawal of inotropic drugs if possible, treatment of fever, and optimization of sedation and hemodynamics (see Chapter 31). The best strategy for treatment is a combination of systemic cooling, synchronized pacing, and intravenous amiodarone infusion. Pacing options include atrial pacing at a rate slightly faster than the tachycardia and dual chamber pacing with the atrial and ventricular connections the wrong way round to synchronize the atrium to the tachycardia rate. This should be undertaken cautiously and only by those with experience of temporary epicardial pacing. Early postoperative JET usually runs its course within 3–5 days and treatment can be withdrawn. It may coexist with complete AV block.

Key references

Collins KK, Van Hare GF, Kertesz NJ, et al. Pediatric nonpost-operative junctional ectopic tachycardia medical management and interventional therapies. *J Am Coll Cardiol* 2009;**53**:690–7.

Dodge-Khatami A, Miller OI, Anderson RH, et al. Surgical substrates of postoperative junctional ectopic tachycardia in congenital heart defects. *J Thorac Cardiovasc Surg* 2002;**123**:624–30.

Laird WP, Snyder CS, Kertesz NJ, et al. Use of intravenous amiodarone for postoperative junctional ectopic tachycardia in children. *Pediatr Cardiol* 2003;**24**:133–7.

Janousek J, Vojtovic P, Gebauer RA. Use of a modified, commercially available temporary pacemaker for R wave synchronized atrial pacing in postoperative junctional ectopic tachycardia. *Pacing Clin Electrophysiol* 2003;**26**:579–86.

Mildh L, Hiippala A, Rautiainen P, et al. Junctional ectopic tachycardia after surgery for congenital heart disease: incidence, risk factors and outcome. *Eur J Cardiothorac Surg* 2011;**39**:75–80.

Sarubbi B, Musto B, Ducceschi V, et al. Congenital junctional ectopic tachycardia in children and adolescents: a 20 year experience based study. *Heart* 2002;**88**:188–90.

Villain E, Vetter VL, Garcia JM, et al. Evolving concepts in the management of congenital junctional ectopic tachycardia. A multicenter study. *Circulation* 1990;**81**:1544–9.

Walsh EP, Saul JP, Sholler GF, et al. Evaluation of a staged treatment protocol for rapid automatic junctional tachycardia after operation for congenital heart disease. *J Am Coll Cardiol* 1997;**29**:1046–53.

18 Ventricular tachycardia

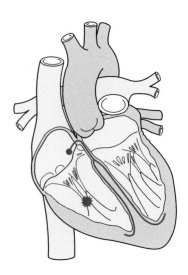

Ventricular tachycardia (VT) is a less common but very important cause of tachycardia in pediatric practice. It is a diagnosis that many pediatricians and some pediatric cardiologists seem reluctant to make, partly because it is perceived to be a universally ominous arrhythmia. VT is frequently misdiagnosed as supraventricular tachycardia (SVT) if the child is not syncopal and is not known to have serious heart disease.

Just as "SVT" is an inadequate final diagnosis and is merely a group name for a variety of arrhythmias that share some common features, so we should not be content with a final diagnosis of VT. There are many different types of VT in infants and children, and in young adults with congenital heart disease. Each has its own etiology, substrate, mechanism, ECG appearance, prognosis, and response to therapy. The various types include neonatal VT (see Chapter 19), incessant idiopathic infant VT (see Chapter 20), idiopathic left ventricular tachycardia (see Chapter 21), idiopathic right ventricular tachycardia (see Chapter 22), congenital long QT syndrome (see Chapter 25), catecholaminergic polymorphic VT (see Chapter 26), and late postoperative VT (see Chapter 32), each of which is dealt with elsewhere. This chapter considers some generic features of VT.

ECG diagnosis

VT is defined as an arrhythmia with three or more consecutive beats originating in the ventricles usually at a rate of 120/min or more (the lower limit is 100/min in adults). The same arrhythmia with a lower ventricular rate is called idioventricular rhythm. On the surface ECG, the QRS has a different shape from, and is wider than, the normal QRS in sinus rhythm. Bear in mind that in some cases the QRS may not be wider than the normal range for age, and in some neonates is less than 100 ms. The two examples in Figure 18.1 and 18.2, both from neonates, illustrate the range – the first in Figure 18.1 had idiopathic neonatal VT (see Chapter 19) and the second in Figure 18.2 had hyperkalemia.

Concise Guide to Pediatric Arrhythmias, First Edition. Christopher Wren.
© 2012 John Wiley & Sons, Ltd. Published 2012 by John Wiley & Sons, Ltd.

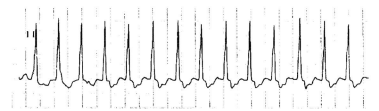

Figure 18.1

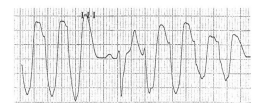

Figure 18.2

An episode of VT is described as sustained if it lasts for more than 30 s and non-sustained if less. VT can also be described as either monomorphic, meaning that it has a constant appearance (QRS shape, axis, etc.), or polymorphic. Most VT is monomorphic. Polymorphic VT is seen in the long QT syndrome (see Chapter 25) and catecholaminergic polymorphic VT (see Chapter 26).

The example in Figure 18.3 shows an 11-beat run of non-sustained monomorphic VT. It also illustrates a common and very helpful feature, ventriculoatrial dissociation. Arrows indicate the position of the P waves and show that sinus rhythm continues in the atrium, unaffected by the VT.

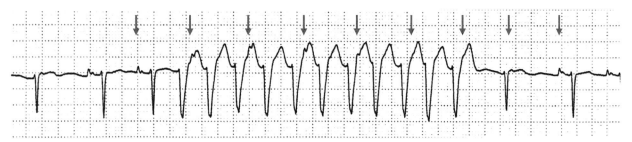

Figure 18.3

Figure 18.4 shows another example, from an 11 year old with an apparent dilated cardiomyopathy. There is a sustained tachycardia with a slightly widened QRS. The QRS complexes are regular and slower dissociated P waves are clearly seen (arrows).

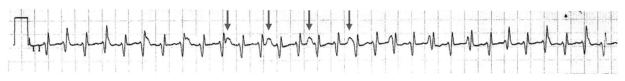

Figure 18.4

Most VT in children occurs with dissociated P waves (retrograde block), particularly at high ventricular rates, but they are not always easy to see. In Figure 18.5, with a rhythm strip from lead V1, the ventricular rate is high, making P waves particularly hard to identify. However, irregularities in the height and shape of the T waves (red arrows) strongly suggest atrial dissociation.

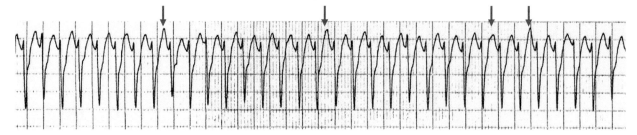

Figure 18.5

There may be other evidence of ventriculoatrial (VA) dissociation. Fusion beats and capture beats may be seen at lower ventricular rates. A sinus capture beat produces an early normal QRS if the preceding P wave arrives at just the right time. In the ECG in Figure 18.6, from a neonate, there is initially 1:1 retrograde conduction with a P wave just after each QRS (black arrow). When retrograde conduction fails there is no retrograde P wave and the subsequent sinus P wave is conducted anterogradely, producing a capture beat that is slightly earlier than the next VT beat would have been and has a normal QRS (first red arrow). Subsequent dissociated P waves are obvious.

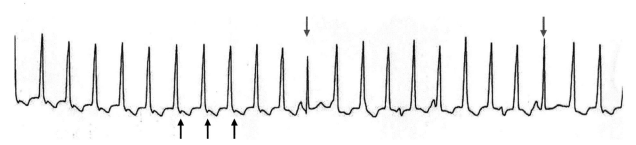

Figure 18.6

A fusion beat is similar to a capture beat but gives a QRS morphology that is a hybrid between normal and that seen in VT. In the example in Figure 18.6 there is a fusion beat, with a slightly earlier and narrower QRS (second red arrow). Atrial dissociation may not be seen at rest but is sometimes more obvious after administration of adenosine (see Chapter 6).

Sometimes the tachycardia is so fast and the QRS so wide that there is little prospect of identifying atrial dissociation, as in the example in Figure 18.7 from a 14-year-old boy. He had undergone repair of a ventricular septal defect in infancy but had an otherwise normal heart. The atypical right bundle branch block (RBBB) pattern and the QS pattern in V6 in this example make VT the almost certain diagnosis. Faced with an ECG like this it is best to assume that the diagnosis is VT (and to proceed accordingly) unless proved otherwise.

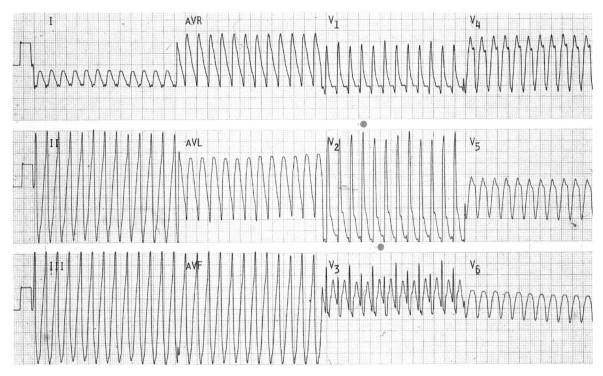

Figure 18.7

The ECG will often give a clue to the origin of the tachycardia. The example in Figure 18.8 shows a 12-lead ECG recording of VT with a QRS pattern more like RBBB than left bundle branch block (LBBB) and a superior axis. This suggests an origin in the posterior part of the left ventricle. There is also clear evidence of VA dissociation.

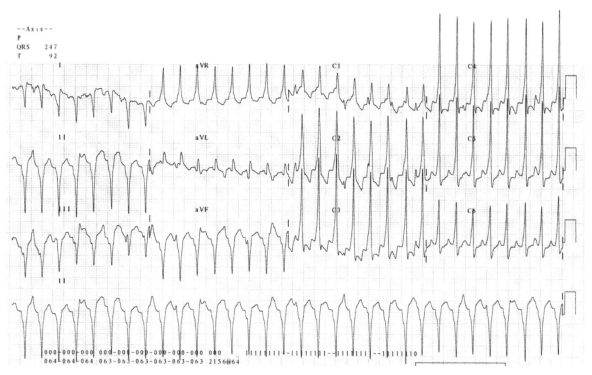

Figure 18.8

The ECG in Figure 18.9 shows VT with a pattern similar to LBBB and an inferior axis, suggesting an origin in the right ventricular outflow.

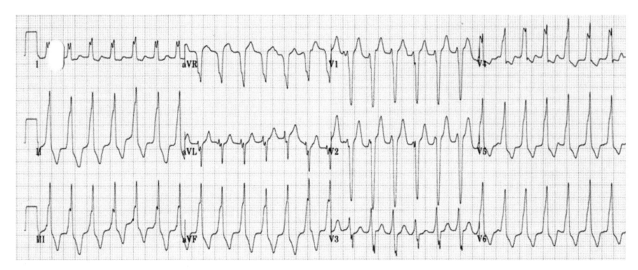

Figure 18.9

Differential diagnosis

The differential diagnosis of VT includes a variety of supraventricular tachycardias. VT originating in the left ventricle, and having an appearance similar to RBBB needs to be distinguished from any SVT with rate-related or pre-existing RBBB and from antidromic AV re-entry with a left-sided accessory pathway. VT originating in the right ventricle, with an appearance similar to LBBB should be distinguished from any supraventricular tachycardia with rate-related or pre-existing LBBB, atriofascicular re-entry tachycardia (see Chapter 15), and antidromic AV re-entry with a right-sided accessory pathway. These features are discussed at more length in Chapter 5.

The role of electrophysiology study

Invasive electrophysiology study is now rarely necessary other than as part of a catheter ablation procedure. However, it may be indicated to establish the diagnosis if a wide QRS tachycardia has been detected on ambulatory monitoring and the mechanism is not known, or for mapping of the arrhythmia before surgery for late postoperative VT.

Presentation and causes

The presentation of VT is just as variable as with SVT, ranging from syncope through heart failure from incessant tachycardia, presyncope, and palpitations, to an incidental finding during monitoring. The many types of VT have many causes, as listed in Table 18.1.

Table 18.1 Acute and chronic causes of ventricular arrhythmias

Acute causes of ventricular arrhythmia		Chronic causes of ventricular arrhythmia	
Metabolic	hypoxia	Congenital	tetralogy of Fallot
	acidemia		coronary abnormalities
	hyperkalemia		mitral valve prolapse
	hypokalemia	Cardiomyopathy	ARVC
	hypocalcemia		hypertrophic cardiomyopathy
	hypomagnesemia		dilated cardiomyopathy
	hypoglycemia	Channelopathy	long QT syndrome
Ischemic	coronary anomalies		CPVT
Traumatic	cardiac surgery		Brugada syndrome
	trauma	Acquired	cardiac tumor
Infective	myocarditis	Postoperative	
	rheumatic fever	Drugs	
Toxic	drugs	Idiopathic	
	poisoning		
	substance abuse		
Idiopathic			

ARVC, arrhythmogenic right ventricular cardiomyopathy; CPVT, catecholaminergic polymorphic ventricular tachycardia.

Acute treatment

The acute treatment of VT depends on the likely cause and clinical situation. In the presence of significant hemodynamic compromise the best option is synchronized DC cardioversion using 1–2 J/kg. If time and the patient's clinical condition allow, intravenous lidocaine 0.5–1.0 mg/kg by injection (followed if necessary by 0.6–3.0 mg/kg/h by infusion) may be used. If there is a primary metabolic cause this must be corrected. Specific types of VT discussed elsewhere may respond to intravenous β-blocker or verapamil. Difficult early postoperative VT related to impaired ventricular function may respond to administration of magnesium sulfate 0.1–0.2 mmol/kg (25–50 mg/kg).

Longer-term management

The management plan depends on the specific type of VT and its cause and is considered in detail elsewhere. Options include no treatment (if the arrhythmia is judged to be benign and there are no symptoms), antiarrhythmic drugs, catheter ablation, surgery, and defibrillator implantation.

Ventricular tachycardia and a normal heart

There are some children who are found to have VT with no sign of heart disease. Some have typical idiopathic right (see Chapter 21) or left (see Chapter 22) VT but others are difficult to classify. They are usually asymptomatic and their VT is an incidental finding. The arrhythmia is usually non-sustained but can be frequent on ambulatory monitoring. It may be induced at lower levels of exercise but is suppressed at higher levels. It is usually only slightly faster than the sinus rate and is generally unresponsive to medication. The prognosis is benign with few late problems reported but such children merit long-term review.

Ventricular tachycardia in poisoning

VT is occasionally observed in children with accidental or self-poisoning. It occurs in poisoning with tricyclic antidepressants, salicylates, phenothiazines, antihistamines, cocaine, and a variety of antiarrhythmic drugs including digoxin, flecainide, amiodarone. The specific management depends on the responsible agent and guidance will be available from the local poisons advice centre. VT also occurs in a variety of metabolic disturbances, particularly hyperkalemia, as in the example in Figure 18.10. Management in this situation involves urgent reduction in potassium concentration by administration of calcium, glucose and insulin, bicarbonate, etc.

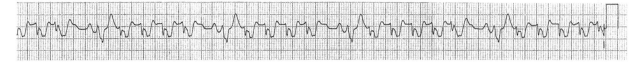

Figure 18.10

Key references

Kugler J. Intention to treat: To the heart of the matter for young patients with ventricular tachycardia. *Heart Rhythm* 2004;**1**:309–10.

Pfammatter JP, Bauersfeld U. Idiopathic ventricular tachycardias in infants and children. *Card Electrophysiol Rev* 2002;**6**:88–92.

Song MK, Baek JS, Kwon BS, et al. Clinical spectrum and prognostic factors of pediatric ventricular tachycardia. *Circ J* 2010;**74**:1951–8.

Wang S, Zhu W, Hamilton RM, et al. Diagnosis-specific characteristics of ventricular tachycardia in children with structurally normal hearts. *Heart Rhythm* 2010;**7**:1725–31.

19   Neonatal ventricular tachycardia

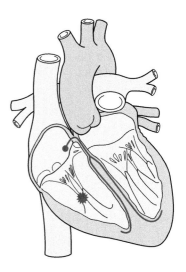

Ventricular tachycardia is a rare arrhythmia in newborn babies, although it may be more common than we appreciate. The diagnosis might easily be overlooked, as the ventricular rate is often only a little faster than sinus rhythm. As a result of this babies are usually asymptomatic.

ECG diagnosis

The QRS complexes are wider than normal for age but the widening is often subtle. The ECG usually shows a pattern resembling partial left bundle branch block, suggesting a tachycardia origin in the right ventricle. As the rate of the tachycardia is usually only a little faster than sinus rhythm there is often 1:1 ventriculoatrial conduction with retrogradely conducted P waves (black arrows in Figure 19.1).

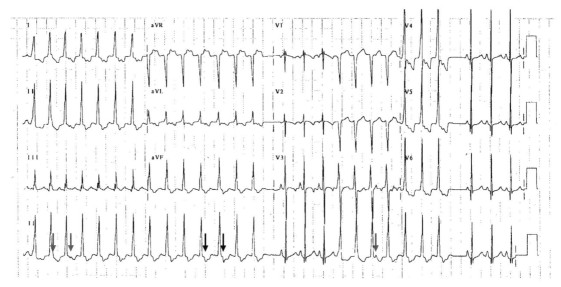

Figure 19.1

Concise Guide to Pediatric Arrhythmias, First Edition. Christopher Wren.
© 2012 John Wiley & Sons, Ltd. Published 2012 by John Wiley & Sons, Ltd.

Sometimes the P waves are dissociated and the finding of a wide QRS tachycardia with retrograde block confirms the diagnosis of ventricular tachycardia. In the example in Figure 19.1, dissociated P waves are clearly seen in the lead II rhythm strip (red arrows) as well as in other leads. The tachycardia is intermittent and the narrowness of the QRS in sinus beats can be compared with the wider QRS in tachycardia.

In the example in Figure 19.2, from a different baby, the appearance of the QRS is very similar. The retrograde P waves are earlier and less obvious although still clear when looked for (black arrows). Tachycardia breaks transiently to reveal a normal QRS in sinus rhythm. When it restarts the P waves are dissociated (red arrow).

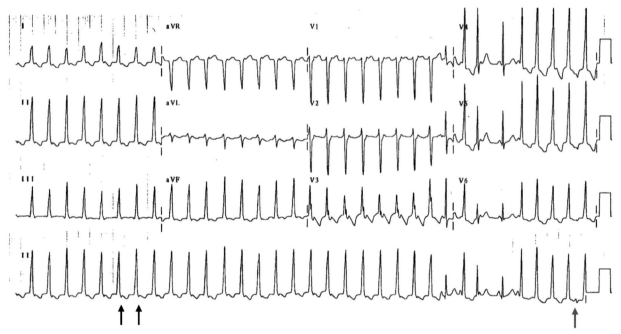

Figure 19.2

Figure 19.3 shows an enlarged view of the ECG in Figure 19.2 and the contrast between the normal and wider QRS is more easily appreciated. The P waves are regular – not all can be seen as some are hidden behind QRS complexes but the ventriculoatrial (VA) dissociation is clear.

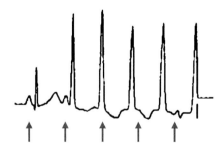

Figure 19.3

In Figure 19.4 there is sinus rhythm alternating with short runs of ventricular tachycardia. The QRS morphology is similar to the two cases above but with a slightly different appearance, which makes prediction of the site of origin of the tachycardia more difficult.

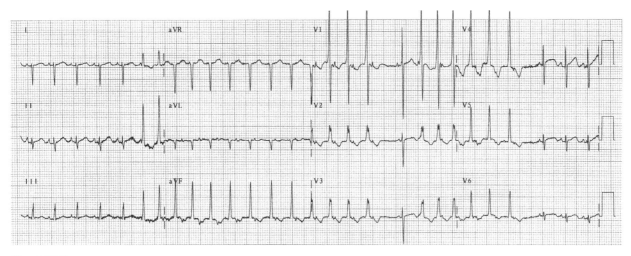

Figure 19.4

The rhythm strip in Figure 19.5 shows a short episode of ventricular tachycardia. There is VA dissociation for the first two beats and the third and subsequent QRS complexes are all followed by P waves (arrows). Tachycardia stops spontaneously and is followed by sinus rhythm.

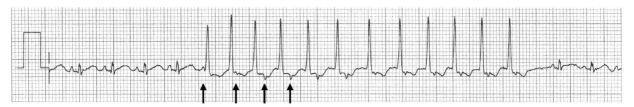

Figure 19.5

If there is consistent 1:1 retrograde conduction leading to doubt about the diagnosis on ECG, intravenous adenosine will help. Adenosine will not stop the tachycardia but will produce VA dissociation (see Chapter 6).

Treatment

Neonates with this type of ventricular tachycardia often do not require treatment. If the baby is asymptomatic and the average heart rate over 24-hour monitoring is not much above normal, then no medication is needed. If tachycardia is more or less incessant and significantly faster than sinus rhythm, treatment with a β-blocker will usually be effective. Amiodarone is occasionally required for resistant cases. The tachycardia usually resolves within weeks and late recurrence is rare.

Key references

Davis A, Gow RM, McCrindle BW, et al. Clinical spectrum, therapeutic management, and follow-up of ventricular tachycardia in infants and young children. *Am Heart J* 1996;**131**:186–91.

Levin MD, Stephens P, Tanel RE, et al. Ventricular tachycardia in infants with structurally normal heart: a benign disorder. *Cardiol Young* 2010;**20**:641–7.

Perry JC. Ventricular tachycardia in neonates. *Pacing Clin Electrophysiol* 1997;**20**:2061–4.

Pfammatter JP, Paul T. Idiopathic ventricular tachycardia in infancy and childhood: a multicenter study on clinical profile and outcome. *J Am Coll Cardiol* 1999;**33**:2067–72.

Villain E, Butera G, Bonnet D, et al. Neonatal ventricular tachycardia. *Arch Mal Coeur Vaiss* 1998;**91**:623–9.

20   Incessant idiopathic infant ventricular tachycardia

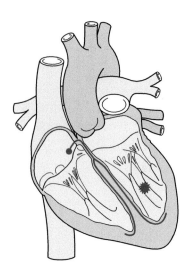

Incessant idopathic infant ventricular tachycardia is a rare arrhythmia that usually presents at between 3 months and 2 years of age. The diagnosis may be overlooked initially and in the past it has often been mistaken for a supraventricular tachycardia. The reported ventricular rates range from 170/min to 440/min with a mean of 260/min. It is more common in boys. "Incessant" is defined as being present for more than 10% of the time but tachycardia is usually constant, and on presentation there is usually evidence of poor ventricular function. The underlying cause in most cases is probably a microscopic posterior left ventricular tumor ("myocardial hamartoma") too small to be seen on echocardiography.

ECG diagnosis

The ECG usually shows a type of right bundle branch block morphology and a superior axis predicting an origin in the posterior or inferior left ventricle (see below). There is usually clear evidence of ventriculoatrial (VA) block with dissociated P waves, or capture beats or fusion beats. The finding of a wide QRS tachycardia with retrograde block confirms the diagnosis of ventricular tachycardia. In the ECG in Figure 20.1 dissociated P waves are clearly seen in the lead II rhythm strip (red arrows) as well as in other leads. The QRS has a notably slurred onset.

Concise Guide to Pediatric Arrhythmias, First Edition. Christopher Wren.
© 2012 John Wiley & Sons, Ltd. Published 2012 by John Wiley & Sons, Ltd.

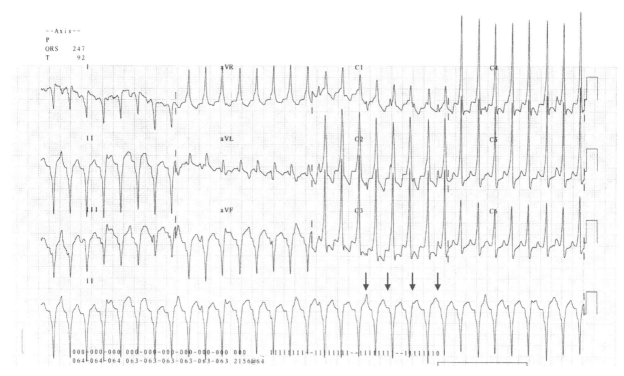

Figure 20.1

In Figure 20.2 the QRS has a right bundle branch block pattern with a sharp upstroke, perhaps suggesting a tachycardia origin within or close to the Purkinje system. The dissociated P waves are less evident although still evident when looked for – they are best seen as an irregularity in the shape of the T waves (red arrows).

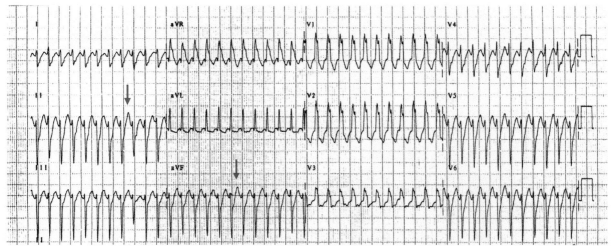

Figure 20.2

In the ECG in Figure 20.3 the QRS is very wide with a slurred upstroke, perhaps indicating an origin within working myocardium. Dissociated P waves are very clear (red arrows), and there is a fusion beat (black arrow) caused by a P wave being conducted to the ventricles and producing an earlier and more normal QRS.

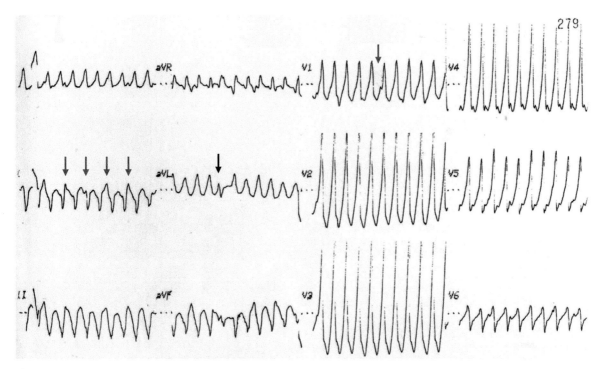

Figure 20.3

If there is any doubt about the diagnosis on ECG, administration of intravenous adenosine will help. Adenosine will not stop the tachycardia but should unmask or accentuate evidence of VA dissociation.

Treatment

Immediate treatment involves control of tachycardia and general support or resuscitation as required. Intravenous lidocaine 1–2 mg/kg will usually slow or stop the tachycardia, leading to a rapid symptomatic improvement. Intravenous amiodarone is an alternative. Incessant idiopathic infant ventricular tachycardia was initially reported to respond poorly to drug treatment but more recent experience is that drugs such as amiodarone and flecainide are usually effective in controlling the arrhythmia, sometimes in combination with a β-blocker. The tachycardia usually resolves before the age of 5 years and drug treatment can then be withdrawn. Late recurrence is unusual.

Key references

Davis A, Gow RM, McCrindle BW, et al. Clinical spectrum, therapeutic management, and follow-up of ventricular tachycardia in infants and young children. *Am Heart J* 1996;**131**:186–91.

Garson A Jr, Smith RT Jr, Moak DL, et al. Incessant ventricular tachycardia in infants: myocardial hamartomas and surgical cure. *J Am Coll Cardiol* 1987;**10**:619–26.

Perry JC. Ventricular tachycardia in neonates. *Pacing Clin Electrophysiol* 1997;**20**:2061–4.

Pfammatter JP, Paul T. Idiopathic ventricular tachycardia in infancy and childhood: a multicenter study on clinical profile and outcome. *J Am Coll Cardiol* 1999;**33**:2067–72.

Thiagalingam A, Winlaw D, Hejmadi A, et al. Images in cardiovascular medicine. Incessant ventricular tachycardia in an infant treated with transmural radiofrequency ablation. *Circulation* 2002;**105**:2797.

Villain E, Bonnet D, Kachaner J, et al. Tachycardies ventriculaires incessantes idiopathiques du nourrisson. *Arch Mal Coeur Vaiss* 1990;**83**:665–71.

Villain E, Butera G, Bonnet D, et al. Neonatal ventricular tachycardia. *Arch Mal Coeur Vaiss* 1998;**91**:623–9.

Idiopathic left ventricular tachycardia

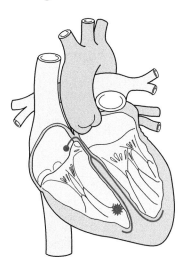

Idiopathic left ventricular tachycardia is a rare arrhythmia. It affects teenagers and young adults and is more common in boys than girls. It presents with symptoms (palpitations, dizziness, dyspnea or presyncope) which may occur at rest but are often triggered by exertion or excitement.

Idiopathic left ventricular tachycardia is also known as left posterior fascicular tachycardia because it is thought to originate in the Purkinje system, low on the left ventricular side of the septum, in the region of the posterior fascicle of the left bundle branch. Other types of idiopathic left ventricular tachycardia are reported but are very rare

ECG diagnosis

The ECG in sinus rhythm is normal. In tachycardia there is a right bundle branch block (RBBB) pattern with a leftward or superior QRS axis. In the example in Figure 21.1, from a 13-year-old girl, the ventricular rate is 160/min and the QRS

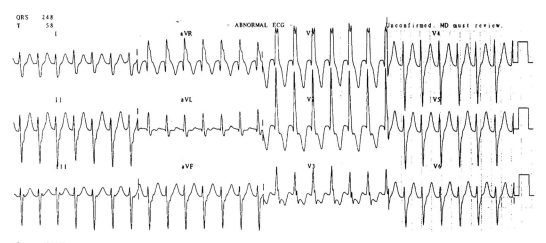

Figure 21.1

complexes show a RBBB-like pattern, with a slightly taller initial component to the R wave, and the mean frontal axis is around −90°. Note the very sharp upstroke of the QRS, suggesting an origin within specialized conduction tissue rather than within working myocardium. P waves are not visible so the diagnosis of ventricular tachycardia is suspected but not proven from this recording.

The example in Figure 21.2 is technically poor, having been through a fax machine, but it does show the consistency of the ECG appearances. There is a superior axis and the R′ is slightly taller than the initial R in V1.

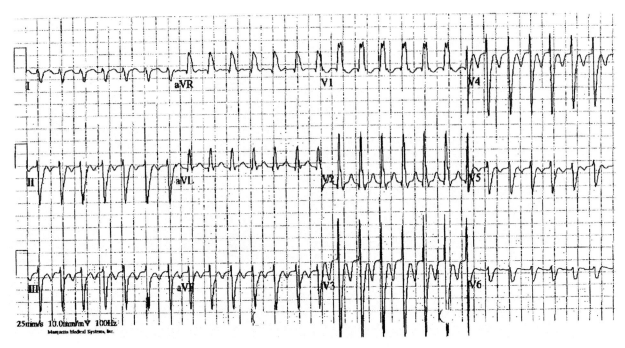

Figure 21.2

Another example of posterior fascicular ventricular tachycardia (VT) is shown in Figure 21.3 with a very similar appearance to those above. The ventricular rate is 175/min, the initial component of the R wave in V1 is taller than the second, and the mean frontal QRS axis is around −120°.

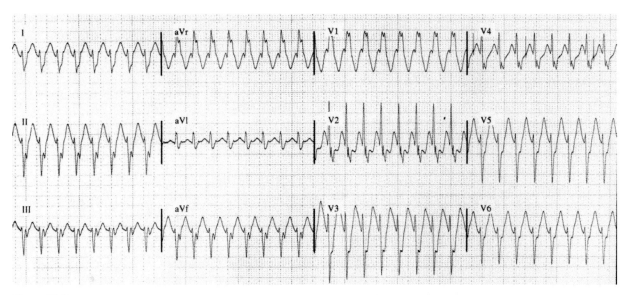

Figure 21.3

The differential diagnosis includes other tachycardias with an RBBB pattern, i.e. any supraventricular tachycardia (SVT) with pre-existing or rate-related RBBB and antidromic atrioventricular (AV) re-entry with a left-sided accessory pathway (see Chapter 5). The ECG appearances are similar to those seen in incessant infant VT, which also usually shows an RBBB pattern with a leftward or superior QRS axis, and probably originates in the inferior or posterior part of the left ventricle (see Chapter 20). However, this type of infant VT is characteristically incessant and behaves more like an automatic or ectopic focal arrhythmia.

Left posterior fascicular tachycardia is a benign form of VT and occurs in the absence of structural heart disease. The echocardiogram will be normal except in rare cases where incessant tachycardia may be associated with impaired ventricular function. Decisions about treatment are based on the symptoms. Acute termination usually cannot be achieved with adenosine and is unreliable with an intravenous β-blocker. Intravenous verapamil is usually effective.

Treatment

Oral treatment with drugs can be used and again verapamil is said to be the most effective, although the response may be variable. An oral β-blocker is an alternative. However, episodes of tachycardia are relatively infrequent in symptomatic patients, and many doses of verapamil will be needed for prevention of one episode of VT.

For most patients the long-term treatment of choice is catheter ablation. Most series report a success rate of around 80%, although the arrhythmia can be difficult to induce at electrophysiology study. The target for ablation may be identified by pace mapping or by recording early systolic or presystolic potentials.

Key references

Arya A, Haghjoo M, Emkanjoo Z, et al. Comparison of presystolic Purkinje and late diastolic potentials for selection of ablation site in idiopathic verapamil sensitive left ventricular tachycardia. *J Interv Card Electrophysiol* 2004;**11**:135–41.

Belhassen B, Shapira I, Pelleg A, et al. Idiopathic recurrent sustained ventricular tachycardia responsive to verapamil: an ECG-electrophysiologic entity. *Am Heart J* 1984;**108**:1034–7.

Ouyang F, Cappato R, Ernst S, et al. Electroanatomic substrate of idiopathic left ventricular tachycardia: unidirectional block and macroreentry within the Purkinje network. *Circulation* 2002;**105**:462–9.

Pfammatter JP, Paul T. Idiopathic ventricular tachycardia in infancy and childhood: a multicenter study on clinical profile and outcome. *J Am Coll Cardiol* 1999;**33**:2067–72.

Ramprakash B, Jaishankar S, Rao HB, et al. Catheter ablation of fascicular ventricular tachycardia. *Indian Pacing Electrophysiol J* 2008;**8**:193–201.

Stevenson WG, Soejima K. Catheter ablation for ventricular tachycardia. *Circulation* 2007;**115**;2750–60.

Yasui K, Shibata T, Yokoyama U, et al. Idiopathic sustained left ventricular tachycardia in pediatric patients. *Pediatr Int* 2001;**43**:42–7.

22 Idiopathic right ventricular tachycardia

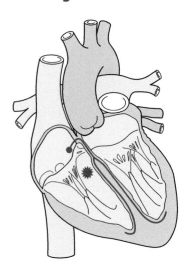

Idiopathic right ventricular tachycardia is an uncommon type of ventricular tachycardia (VT) that usually arises in the right ventricular outflow tract. The anatomical substrate for this arrhythmia is poorly defined but it has an odd electropharmacological profile, which suggests that it may be caused by triggered activity (as opposed to the more common re-entry or automatic arrhythmias). The arrhythmia has a focal origin because it can be abolished by a single application of ablation energy.

ECG diagnosis

Idiopathic right ventricular tachycardia usually comes to notice after an incidental finding of an irregular or high heart rate or abnormal ECG, but sometimes produces symptoms of palpitation or presyncope (only rarely syncope). The ECG in sinus rhythm is normal. The 12-lead ECG or 24-hour ECG may show an intermittent repetitive tachycardia or sustained tachycardia. There is a wide QRS, with a morphology similar to left bundle branch block (LBBB) and an inferior mean frontal QRS axis. It is important to distinguish this from other causes of tachycardia with an LBBB pattern such as supraventricular tachycardias with pre-existing or rate-related LBBB, and antidromic AV re-entry with a right-sided accessory pathway (see Chapter 5).

The ECG in Figure 22.1 comes from a 6-year-old boy with few symptoms despite incessant tachycardia and mildly abnormal ventricular function. The ventricular rate is 170/min and P waves are visible intermittently, giving evidence of ventriculoatrial dissociation (red arrows) and confirming VT. The intervening P waves are hidden by the QRS complexes and T waves. This arrhythmia was abolished by ablation in the right ventricular outflow.

Concise Guide to Pediatric Arrhythmias, First Edition. Christopher Wren.
© 2012 John Wiley & Sons, Ltd. Published 2012 by John Wiley & Sons, Ltd.

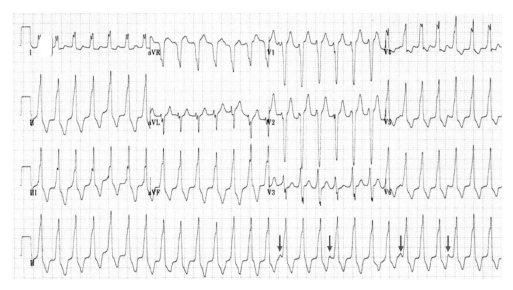

Figure 22.1

The example in Figure 22.2 shows a 24-hour ECG recording from an asymptomatic 7-year-old girl. Recurrent repetitive monomorphic VT is seen with short periods of sinus rhythm in between. The ventricular rate is around 150/min and each run slows slightly just before it stops.

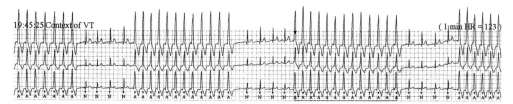

Figure 22.2

Another example of recurrent non-sustained VT is shown in Figure 22.3. Again the QRS complexes have an appearance similar to LBBB with a mean frontal QRS axis of around +75°. Although P waves are not seen during VT, the sinus pause at the end of each run of VT suggests that there is retrograde conduction to the atria with transient sinus suppression.

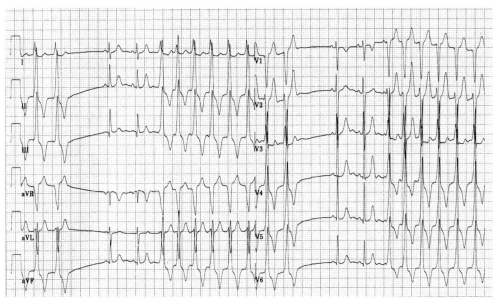

Figure 22.3

The response to exercise in idiopathic right VT is variable but the arrhythmia is often suppressed at high heart rates and workloads. Less commonly it can be precipitated by exertion or emotion.

Idiopathic right VT needs to be distinguished from arrhythmogenic right ventricular cardiomyopathy (ARVC). The latter is rare in childhood and is mainly a disease of young adult males who present with syncope or a family history of sudden death. Patients with ARVC have abnormalities of right ventricular function on magnetic resonance imaging (MRI) or echocardiography which can be subtle. Children presenting with probable idiopathic right VT should have an echocardiogram but will usually not require MRI.

Treatment

Most children with idiopathic right VT probably do not require treatment. The arrhythmia is intrinsically benign and is not associated with a risk of sudden death. Drug treatment, most often with a β-blocker or verapamil, but sometimes with drugs such as amiodarone or flecainide, has been tried but the response is often disappointing and there is no evidence that it offers an improvement over the natural history. Catheter ablation is often effective but is indicated only in the presence of significant symptoms or concern over ventricular function.

Key references

Harris KC, Potts JE, Fournier A, et al. A multicenter study of right ventricular outflow tract tachycardia in children. *J Pediatr* 2006;**149**:822–6.

Kim RJ, Iwai S, Markowitz SM, et al. Clinical and electrophysiological spectrum of idiopathic ventricular outflow tract arrhythmias. *J Am Coll Cardiol* 2007;**49**:2035–43.

O'Donnell D, Cox D, Bourke J, et al. Clinical and electrophysiological differences between patients with arrhythmogenic right ventricular dysplasia and right ventricular outflow tract tachycardia. *Eur Heart J* 2003;**24**:801–10.

Pfammatter JP, Paul T. Idiopathic ventricular tachycardia in infancy and childhood: a multicenter study on clinical profile and outcome. *J Am Coll Cardiol* 1999;**33**:2067–72.

Stevenson WG, Soejima K. Catheter ablation for ventricular tachycardia. *Circulation* 2007;**115**;2750–60.

Tandri H, Bluemke DA, Ferrari VA, et al. Findings on magnetic resonance imaging of idiopathic right ventricular outflow tachycardia. *Am J Cardiol* 2004;**94**:1441–5.

Vaseghi M, Shivkumar K. Catheter ablation of idiopathic ventricular tachycardia. *Circ Arrhythm Electrophysiol* 2010;**3**:3219–21.

23 Ventricular premature beats

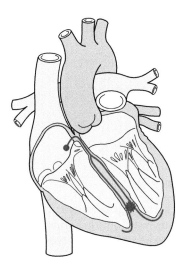

Ventricular premature beats are a common finding in children with normal hearts as well as those with heart disease. Most are benign and very few require treatment.

ECG diagnosis

A ventricular premature beat (also variously described as a premature ventricular contraction or complex, a ventricular ectopic beat, or a ventricular extrasystole) describes an QRS complex that originates earlier than expected from the ventricles. It is recognized by having an abnormal QRS, which is almost always wider than normal and is often similar to a left or right bundle branch block pattern. There is usually no preceding P wave because the next sinus P wave has not yet arrived (black arrow in Figure 23.1 below). If the coupling interval is relatively long, a P wave is sometimes visible.

In the example in Figure 23.1 there is respiratory sinus arrhythmia and a long and variable coupling interval between the ventricular premature beats and the preceding sinus beats. This results in the occasional appearance of a P wave just before the QRS (red arrow) but the P wave is not premature and does not have time to be conducted.

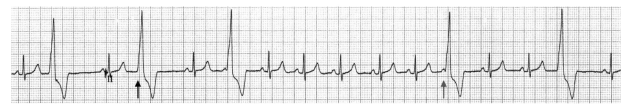

Figure 23.1

Ventricular premature beats sometimes occur in regular patterns. If each alternate beat is premature, this is described as ventricular bigeminy, as in the example in Figure 23.2.

Concise Guide to Pediatric Arrhythmias, First Edition. Christopher Wren.
© 2012 John Wiley & Sons, Ltd. Published 2012 by John Wiley & Sons, Ltd.

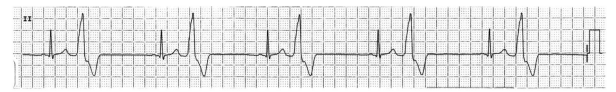

Figure 23.2

If every third beat is premature this is trigeminy (Figure 23.3).

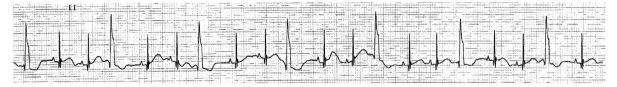

Figure 23.3

Ventricular premature beats may occur in twos – described as pairs or couplets. Couplets are rare in normal children. In the example in Figure 23.4, from a 7-year old boy with late rejection after heart transplantation, there are very frequent ventricular couplets. Although they are usually benign, in this instance they were a marker of a significant myocardial problem.

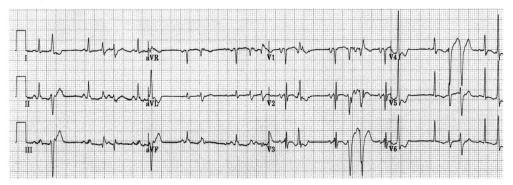

Figure 23.4

Three or more consecutive ventricular premature beats at a rate above 120/min are defined as ventricular tachycardia (see Chapter 18).

The morphology of a ventricular premature beat will give a clue to its site of origin. If it arises in the right ventricle it will resemble left bundle branch block, as in the example in Figure 23.5. These premature beats also show an inferior axis suggesting an origin in the right ventricular outflow.

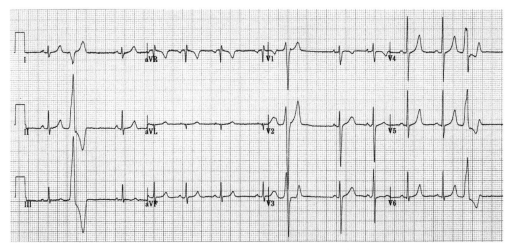

Figure 23.5

In most cases all the ventricular premature beats are the same shape – known as monomorphic or uniform. Much less commonly ventricular premature beats have varying shapes – called polymorphic or multiform. These are unusual in normal hearts.

Ventricular premature beats are usually idiopathic. In an acute setting they may be related to biochemical disturbances such as hypokalemia, acidemia, or hypoxemia. They may be seen in myocarditis or other causes of myocardial damage. They may be caused by mechanical interference from intravenous catheters, etc. They can be caused by drugs and other agents such as caffeine and nicotine.

Almost all ventricular premature beats are benign. They are most often discovered by chance, on an ECG monitored or recorded for another reason. If ventricular premature beats occur in an acute setting (e.g. after cardiac surgery), it is worth checking that serum biochemistry is normal and that there is no mechanical cause (such as a malpositioned monitoring catheter). Investigation of chronic ventricular premature beats should include a 12-lead ECG (which should be otherwise normal). If the beats are frequent, or their discovery causes anxiety, other investigations may include an echocardiogram, and ambulatory and/or exercise ECG. Ventricular premature beats in children with normal hearts are usually suppressed on exercise. The diurnal pattern on ambulatory monitoring is more variable. If they are a chance finding and there are no associated symptoms, no further investigation will be required. If they occur in the context of repaired congenital heart disease they may be kept under review by occasional repeat monitoring. Even then they are unlikely to be very significant. We know, for example, that ventricular premature beats are very common late after repair of a tetralogy of Fallot but are not a predictor of late problems.

Treatment

Treatment of ventricular premature beats is not often indicated. Where a trial of medication is required it may be preferable to start with a β-blocker rather than drugs such as flecainide or amiodarone. Catheter ablation of ventricular premature beats arising in the right ventricular outflow has been reported but is rarely indicated.

Key references

Alexander ME, Berul CI. Ventricular arrhythmias: when to worry. *Pediatr Cardiol* 2000;**21**:532–41.

Jacobsen JR, Garson A Jr, Gillette PC, et al. Premature ventricular contractions in normal children. *J Pediatr* 1978;**92**:36–8.

Paul T, Marchal C, Garson A Jr. Ventricular couplets in the young: prognosis related to underlying substrate. *Am Heart J* 1990;**119**:577–82.

Tsuji A, Nagashima M, Hasegawa S, et al. Long-term follow-up of idiopathic ventricular arrhythmias in otherwise normal children. *Jpn Circ J* 1995;**59**:654–62.

24 Ventricular fibrillation

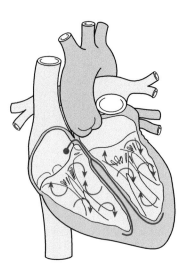

Ventricular fibrillation is defined as turbulent, disorganized, electrical activity of the heart producing ECG deflections that continuously change in shape, magnitude, and direction. It is the most immediately dangerous arrhythmia and produces cardiac arrest. It is a rare arrhythmia in children and is an uncommon cause of out-of-hospital or in-hospital cardiac arrest. Ventricular fibrillation is recognized on the ECG which shows chaotically irregular deflections of variable amplitude with no recognizable QRS complexes. (A similar appearance can be produced by disconnected monitoring leads so it is important to confirm that the patient is unconscious and pulseless.)

Ventricular fibrillation in children is rare. Most of the causes below usually present in a less dramatic way. If resuscitation is successful, extensive investigation will be required to determine the cause.

The causes of ventricular fibrillation

The causes in children include the following:
- Long QT syndrome
- Catecholaminergic polymorphic ventricular tachycardia
- Wolff–Parkinson–White syndrome
- Brugada syndrome
- Cardiomyopathy, including hypertrophic, dilated, and arrhythmogenic right ventricular cardiomyopathies
- Commotio cordis
- Anomalous origin of a coronary artery
- Hypoxia
- Electrocution
- Severe hypothermia
- Drugs: cocaine, glue sniffing, tricyclic antidepressant poisoning
- Severe hyperkalemia
- Cardiac surgery
- Idiopathic.

Concise Guide to Pediatric Arrhythmias, First Edition. Christopher Wren.
© 2012 John Wiley & Sons, Ltd. Published 2012 by John Wiley & Sons, Ltd.

The recording in Figure 24.1 comes from an 11-month-old girl who had an out-of-hospital cardiac arrest. She was successfully resuscitated at hospital but suffered serious long-term brain damage. Despite extensive investigation, no cause was found and there has been no recurrence in more than 13 years of follow-up.

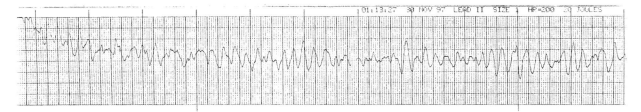

Figure 24.1

Figure 24.2 shows an unusual 12-lead ECG of ventricular fibrillation. This was recorded in a 12-year-old girl with a previous Mustard operation undergoing surgical baffle revision and map-guided surgery for incisional atrial tachycardia. The ventricular fibrillation was produced by systemic hypothermia on cardiopulmonary bypass before cardioplegia was given.

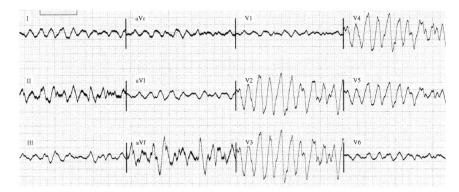

Figure 24.2

The ECG rhythm strip in Figure 24.3 comes from a 16-year-old girl with known, but previously asymptomatic, Wolff–Parkinson–White syndrome. She attended her local hospital emergency department after the sudden onset of palpitations. The upper trace shows her ECG on presentation which was interpreted as "supraventricular tachycardia," but which is an irregular wide QRS tachycardia and is obviously

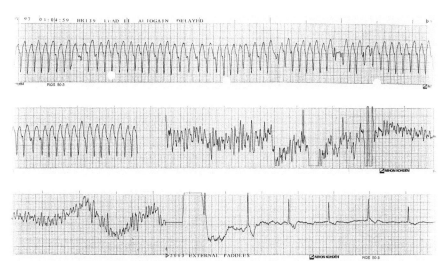

Figure 24.3

pre-excited atrial fibrillation (see Chapter 13). She was treated with intravenous verapamil, which produced ventricular fibrillation (middle trace). Fortunately, this was recognized promptly and she was successfully defibrillated into sinus rhythm. She went on to have an effective radiofrequency ablation.

Treatment

Treatment of ventricular fibrillation follows the guidelines published by the American Heart Association in 2005. Cardiopulmonary resuscitation is started immediately and an unsynchronized shock of 2 J/kg is given as soon as possible. Resuscitation is continued and, if a reasonable rhythm with good cardiac output is not restored immediately, a second shock of 4 J/kg is given. If this does not work, give intravenous epinephrine 0.01 mg/kg (0.1 ml/kg of 1:10 000). Continue chest compressions and repeat the DC shock and epinephrine as necessary. If ventricular fibrillation continues, give amiodarone 5 mg/kg or lidocaine 1 mg/kg. If defibrillation is successful but ventricular fibrillation recurs, continue chest compressions, then give another bolus of amiodarone, and try to defibrillate with the previously successful DC shock dose. Once sinus rhythm, or other rhythm with cardiac output, is restored, search for and correct the underlying cause of the ventricular fibrillation.

Once the cause of the ventricular fibrillation has been determined, further treatment may be required. This may involve definitive cure (e.g. ablation of Wolff–Parkinson–White syndrome), or long-term drug treatment with or without defibrillator implantation.

Key references

ACC/AHA/HRS 2008. Guidelines for device-based therapy of cardiac rhythm abnormalities: Executive summary: A report of the American College of Cardiology/American Heart Association Task Force on Practice Guidelines. *Circulation* 2008;**117**:2820–40.

American Heart Association. Guidelines for cardiopulmonary resuscitation and emergency cardiovascular care. Part 12: Pediatric advanced life support. *Circulation* 2005;**112**:IV-167–87.

Quan L, Franklin WH, eds. *Ventricular Fibrillation: A Pediatric Problem.* NY: Futura Publishing Co Inc. Armonk, 2000.

Samson RA, Nadkarni VM, Meaney PA, et al. Outcomes of in-hospital ventricular fibrillation in children. *N Engl J Med* 2006;**354**:2328–39.

Young KD, Gausche-Hill M, McClung CD, et al. A prospective, population-based study of the epidemiology and outcome of out-of-hospital pediatric cardiopulmonary arrest. *Pediatrics* 2004;**114**:157–64.

25 Long QT syndrome

Congenital long QT syndrome (LQTS) was first described as an association of syncope, sudden death, QT prolongation, and deafness with autosomal recessive inheritance by Jervell and Lange-Nielsen in 1957. A more common form with autosomal dominant inheritance and normal hearing was described independently by Romano and Ward in 1963–4. Since then our understanding of the condition has advanced considerably. The protective effect of β-blocker therapy was reported in the 1970s and the first report of an underlying causative gene mutation came in the 1990s.

Congenital LQTS is now known to be an inherited abnormality of function of ion channels that control sodium and potassium flow through the myocyte cell membrane, and is often referred to as a channelopathy. It is characterized by syncope (caused by polymorphic ventricular tachycardia) and sudden death, associated with prolongation of the Q–T interval on the ECG. The population prevalence of the disease has been estimated at 1:5000 but variable penetrance makes precise assessment difficult.

A causative genetic mutation can now be identified in around 70% of patients with LQTS (up to 90% in familial cases and as low as 30% in isolated cases). LQT1 is caused by a mutation in the *KCNQ1* gene. LQT2 is caused by a mutation in the *KCNH2* gene (also known as *HERG*). LQT3 is caused by a mutation in the sodium channel gene *SCN5A*. Several other gene mutations are known to cause LQTS subtypes 4–13, all of which are rare. Mutations underlying the 30% of cases without an identified cause remain to be discovered. Jervell–Lange-Nielsen syndrome is rare and is mostly caused by a *KCNQ1* mutation.

LQTS is a disease of young people, with almost all of those with symptoms being under 40. Retrospective diagnosis may be made in asymptomatic older family members.

Measurement of the QT interval

Recognition of LQTS depends on accurate measurement of the QT interval. It is measured on a standard 12-lead ECG, usually in lead II and/or lead V5. because these leads usually have an upright T wave with a distinct end. Identifying the onset of the QRS complex is usually easy but the end of the T wave can sometimes be difficult.

The QT interval varies with heart rate, becoming shorter at higher heart rates. As a result of this it is customary to "correct" the measured QT by normalizing it to a heart rate of 60/min, usually by using Bazett's formula:

$$QTc = QT \div \sqrt{RR}$$

The Bazett formula has its limitations but is the only one in general use because it can be performed on a calculator. It becomes less reliable at higher heart rates, such as are often encountered in infants and children.

The QT interval can be measured in seconds or milliseconds but the RR interval is measured in seconds. The RR interval is measured as an average over 5–10 cycles. In the example in Figure 25.1 the QT interval measures 620 ms (red lines). The heart

Concise Guide to Pediatric Arrhythmias, First Edition. Christopher Wren.
© 2012 John Wiley & Sons, Ltd. Published 2012 by John Wiley & Sons, Ltd.

rate averages 55/min, giving an R–R interval of 1.1 s so the rate-corrected QTc is $620 \div \sqrt{1.1} = 591$ ms.

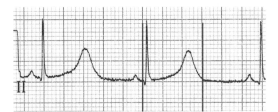

Figure 25.1

A QTc measurement of <440 ms (0.44 s) is generally regarded as normal and values over 460–470 ms (0.46–0.47 s) are abnormal. A measurement of 440–460/470 is borderline and cannot, by itself, confirm or exclude an abnormality. The machine-measured QTc interval is generally reliable but should always be checked by manual measurement when it gives a borderline result or when the diagnosis of LQTS is being considered seriously.

Diagnosis

Although LQTS is a genetic disease, genetic analysis takes some time so diagnosis of LQTS depends on the history and ECG findings. Often the QT prolongation on the ECG is marked and diagnosis is straightforward. In cases of doubt a scoring system may be helpful but it does not resolve all diagnostic difficulty. It was proposed in 1993 and, as far as I am aware, has not been superseded.

The score awards 2 points for syncope under stress, 1 point for syncope without stress and $^1/_2$ point for congenital deafness. There is a score of 1 point for a family member with proven long QT syndrome and $^1/_2$ point for unexplained sudden cardiac death in a first degree relative younger than 30 years.

On the ECG there are 3 points if the QTc is >480ms, 2 points if it is 460–470 ms (I presume this should have been 460–480ms), and 1 point if it is 450–459 in males. The presence of torsades de pointes scores 2 points (but then there cannot also be a score for syncope) but 0 in a patient taking a drug known to cause QT prolongation. T wave alternans (see below) scores 1 point, the presence of notched T waves (but this is not defined) in three separate leads scores 1 point and bradycardia for age scores 1 point (but only in children).

The possible score ranges from zero to a maximum of 9 points. The score is translated into one of three probability categories: 0-1 point gives a low probability of long QT syndrome; 2–3 points an intermediate probability; and 4 or more points a high probability. The authors of the scoring system pointed out that because the Bazett formula for QTc overcorrects at higher heart rates additional caution over the diagnosis is needed when dealing with a patient with sinus tachycardia – as is commonly the case in children.

With an intermediate score of 2–3 points based only on the initial ECG measurement of the QT interval (i.e. the diagnosis cannot be confirmed or ruled out) it is best to record serial ECGs although little is known about the long-term temporal variability of QTc measurements, either in long QT syndrome patients or in normal children. Children in whom the diagnosis cannot be confirmed or excluded certainly deserve to be followed in the clinic. They may also benefit from occasional repeat ambulatory ECG recording and/or exercise testing.

LQTS usually comes to notice through presentation with syncope, presyncope, palpitations, or cardiac arrest, with a family history of sudden death, or through family screening. The diagnosis is sometimes made when an ECG is obtained in an asymptomatic child for another reason. Syncope in LQTS is usually unheralded and often related to exertion and/or excitement. Syncope related to swimming seems particularly common in children with LQT1. Some patients have had many episodes of syncope before a diagnosis is made. Questions about the family should include specific inquiry about a history of syncope or sudden death or "epilepsy" (which is sometimes mistakenly diagnosed in LQTS).

If the diagnosis is suspected but not easily confirmed, other information is required. It is helpful to record 12-lead ECGs from all first-degree relatives because, if any is abnormal, it may help diagnosis. Exercise or ambulatory ECG recordings, and the response to an epinephrine bolus or infusion, have all been proposed as methods of helping diagnosis but so far they are not widely accepted as having sufficient diagnostic precision in borderline cases.

As mentioned above, genetic analysis looking for the mutations known to cause LQTS is now available as a clinical tool. About 70% of patients with a definite clinical diagnosis will be found to have one of the recognized mutations. In most series LQT1 accounts for around 45%, LQT2 for 20%, and LQT3 for 5%. Double mutations are found in <5%. Other types of LQTS are rare and genetic analysis for the underlying mutations may be indicated only if they are suspected on clinical grounds. In 30% of patients with LQTS no mutation will be found. This obviously means that genetic analysis is no help in excluding a diagnosis of LQTS but can be used only to confirm a clinical diagnosis. (The exception to this is in analysis of first-degree relatives in a family in which a mutation has already been recognized.)

Gene-specific variations in T-wave morphology have been described. LQT1 Is often associated with a broad-based T wave, LQT2 commonly produces a bifid T wave, and LQT3 typically has a late-onset peaked T wave, as shown in the examples in Figure 25.2. However, these are not precise predictors of the underlying mutation and there are many exceptions.

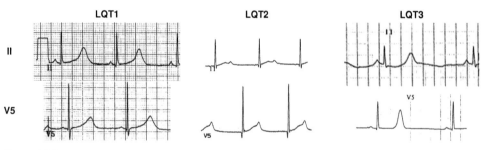

Figure 25.2

The ECG in Figure 25.3 is from a 12-year-old boy with a typical presentation with syncope on exercise and a proven LQT1 mutation. His heart rate is around 55/min and his QT interval is >600 ms. Symptoms are mostly related to exertion in LQT1 and occur at a relatively young age, with 60% of patients experiencing their first symptoms before the age of 10.

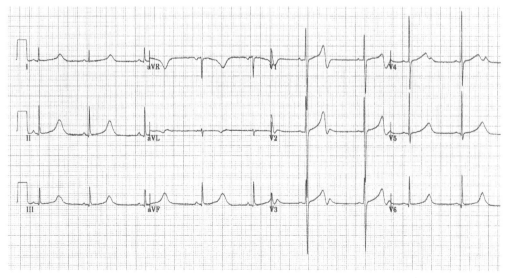

Figure 25.3

An example of LQT2 is shown in Figure 25.4 in a recording from a 10-year-old boy with syncope. Symptoms are less common in LQT2 but the risk of death is probably higher than LQT1. Syncope in LQT2 more often occurs during emotional stress or sleep or at rest.

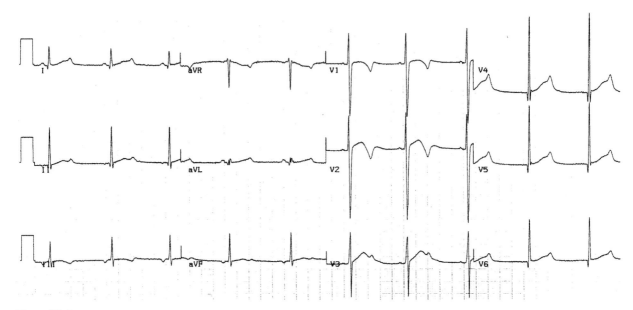

Figure 25.4

The example in Figure 25.5 shows the typical appearance of LQT3 in an 8-year-old boy with mild aortic stenosis who was found by chance to have QT prolongation. The sharply peaked T wave in chest leads follows a long isoelectric ST segment. Symptoms during rest or sleep are also more common than during exercise in LQT3.

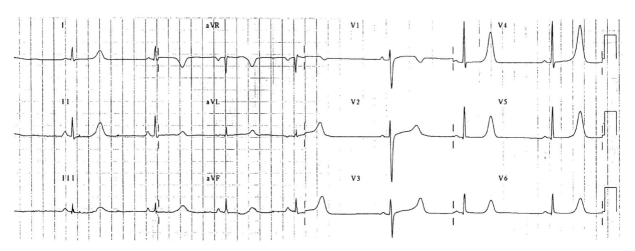

Figure 25.5

The 15-lead ECG in Figure 25.6 comes from a boy with Jervell Lange-Nielsen syndrome. In this rare condition most known patients are symptomatic, presenting with syncope on exercise or during emotional stress at a young age, usually before school age. The QT interval is usually markedly prolonged, as shown here. In this example the T waves are flat in many leads and the QT interval is impossible to measure in leads II and V5, so others leads have to be used.

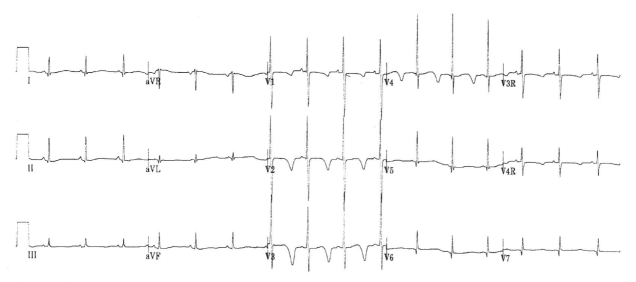

Figure 25.6

T-wave alternans is an uncommon finding. It is associated with marked QT prolongation and is said to be a precursor of torsades de pointes. The recording in Figure 25.7 was made in a 4-year-old boy undergoing transcatheter closure of a patent ductus arteriosus under general anesthetic. His QT prolongation was an incidental finding and he had never had symptoms or arrhythmias. So far his genotype has not been identified.

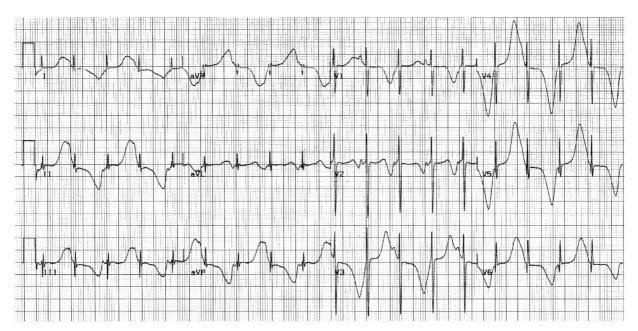

Figure 25.7

The characteristic arrhythmia seen in patients with LQTS is polymorphic ventricular tachycardia, commonly known as torsades de pointes. In most patients with LQTS this arrhythmia is never recorded and it is not necessary for diagnosis. It is mostly seen during prolonged monitoring with Holter recording or on event or loop recording. The ECG shows a rapid irregular sinusoidal activity and varying amplitude with no distinguishable QRS complexes and T waves. Most episodes are self-limiting, as in the example in Figure 25.8.

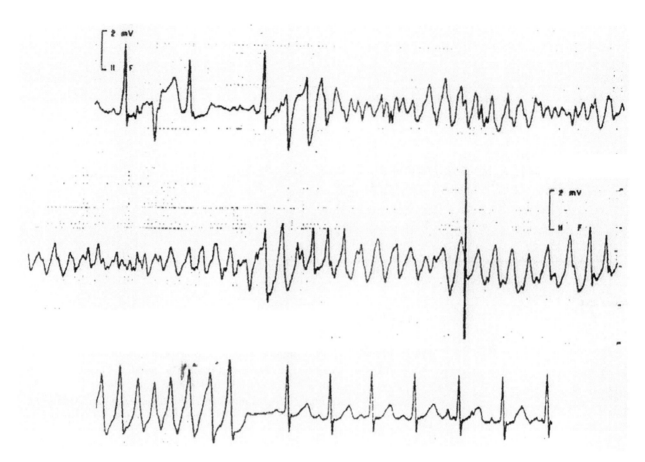

Figure 25.8

Risk stratification

Various predictors of increased risk in LQTS have been described but few of them have a major impact on management. The main predictors of increased risk are a QTc duration of >500 ms and a history of syncope. A family history of premature sudden cardiac death seems not to be independent risk factor.

Management

Management of children with LQTS is complex and consultations early after the diagnosis is suspected or confirmed are often time-consuming. A priority is investigation of other family members, initially limited to first-degree relatives – parents and siblings. As the results of genetic testing will not be available for some time, assessment is based on taking a family history and recording 12-lead ECGs. If any other affected family members are identified in this way, screening may have to be extended.

Confirmation or strong suspicion of the diagnosis will lead to a decision to start treatment, as discussed below. Advice should also be given on limitation of physical activity, particularly avoiding strenuous competitive exercise, and avoidance of drugs known to cause or exacerbate QT prolongation.

There have been no randomized trials of treatment of LQTS so drug treatment strategies are mainly influenced by experience from large centers and international registries. Therapy with a β-blocker is given to almost all patients with LQTS. Nadolol is the drug most often used, in a dose of around 1 mg/kg per day. It has a long half-life and is usually taken once a day. A liquid formulation is available for smaller children. Other β-blockers are also effective, if less convenient. Adequacy of dosing can be confirmed by limitation of the maximum heart rate on exercise testing or ambulatory ECG monitoring. β-Blocker treatment does not shorten the QTc interval, although QTc measurements do vary on repeat recordings during follow-up.

The level of protection offered by β-blocker treatment is high, particularly in LQT1, which is the most common type. Recurrence of syncope or sudden death is usually related to failure of compliance. It is sometimes difficult to assess the results of treatment in large multicenter or registry reports because they may be less certain about compliance than single-centre series. There is some evidence that β-blocker treatment may be less effective in Jervell Lange-Nielsen syndrome.

Pacemaker implantation has been used in some LQT syndrome patients, particularly those with significant bradycardia or LQT3 or Jervell Lange-Nielsen syndrome, but a survival benefit has not been demonstrated.

Recent reports of early experience with genotype-specific drug treatment such as the sodium channel blockers mexiletine and flecainide are interesting but these drugs appear unlikely to replace β-blocker treatment in the near future.

The use of an implantable cardioverter defibrillator (ICD) in LQT syndrome is generally restricted to patients considered to be at high risk, such as those with recurrent syncope despite compliance with β-blocker therapy, and some patients with LQT3 or Jervell Lange-Nielsen syndrome. It may also be recommended if the primary presentation is with resuscitation from cardiac arrest. An ICD is rarely required in LQT1.

Acquired long QT syndrome

Acquired LQTS describes a pathological prolongation of the QT interval on exposure to drugs or in response to other effects and reversion to normal after withdrawal of the stimulus. Such abnormal QT prolongation is associated with polymorphic ventricular tachycardia or ventricular fibrillation, as seen in congenital LQTS. The causes are mostly drugs but also factors such as metabolic disturbances, as listed Table 25.1. The risk of development of acquired LQTS is increased by administration of more than one drug, or use of a drug in the face of other risk factors such as hypokalemia. A full list of drugs associated with a risk of QT prolongation is available on websites such as www.azcert.org.

The risk varies from relatively high (with drugs such as quinidine, dofetilide, and sotalol) to rare, although a low risk may be significant if it is associated with a drug that is widely prescribed. This has led to the withdrawal of drugs such as cisapride and terfenidine and assessing the risk of possible drug-induced QT prolongation is now an important factor in the early development of new drugs. The risk is increased in the face of concurrent administration of another drug on the list or one that inhibits cytochrome P450 drug metabolism.

The common pathway for drug-induced QT prolongation is the inhibition of the delayed rectifier K^+ current, I_{Kr}. This in turn is generated by expression of the gene

Table 25.1 Drugs causing acquired long QT syndrome

Antiarrhythmics, e.g. quinidine, sotalolol, disopyramide
Antihistamines, e.g. terfenidine, astemizole
Macrolide antibiotics, e.g. erythromycin, clarithromycin
Fluoroquinolones, e.g. sparfloxacin, ciprofloxacin
Antimalarials, e.g. chloroquine, halofantine
Imidazole antifungals, e.g. ketoconazole
Tricyclic antidepressants, e.g. imipramine
Antianginals, e.g. bepridil
Prokinetics, e.g. cisapride
Antiemetics, e.g. domperidone, droperidol
Antipsychotics, e.g. haloperidol, thioridazine, pimozide
Anti-infective agents, e.g. pentamidine
Anti-cancer drugs, e.g. arsenic trioxide, tamoxifen

HERG or *KCNH2*, mutations of which cause congenital LQT2. *HERG* channels seem particularly susceptible to drug-induced blockade, a feature thought to be explained by the physical molecular structure of the *HERG* channel. Hypokalemia is a common associated risk factor and has a direct effect on *HERG* function as well as potentiating drug blockade. I_{Kr} blockade and low extracellular K^+ both prolong action potential duration and potentiate development of early after-depolarizations and triggered electric activity, precursors for the development of torsades de pointes. Acquired LQTS may also be potentiated by hypomagnesemia.

The precise underlying cause of acquired LQTS is not as well understood as for congenital LQTS. It seems probable that genetic variation in the activity of enzymes responsible for drug metabolism and polymorphisms in genes known to cause LQTS play some role. A small number of acquired LQTS patients can be shown to have mutations associated with congenital LQTS and may just have a subclinical variant.

Female sex is also a risk factor. QTc intervals are longer in females than males and the risk of ventricular arrhythmias associated with quinidine or sotalol is two or three times higher in females. Females are also more sensitive to I_{Kr}-blocking drugs and have an increased risk of drug-induced torsades de pointes.

There is no threshold level either for the diagnosis of acquired LQTS or for triggering of torsades de pointes. QTc intervals in acquired LQTS are generally very long, >500 ms.

Acute management of acquired LQTS involves withdrawal of the offending agent, correction of hypokalemia to a potassium >4 mmol/L and giving intravenous magnesium. Isoprenaline infusion or temporary pacing may also be useful to prevent any triggering bradycardia or pauses. Further management avoids future avoidance of any positive drug. Acquired LQTS is generally considered not to be familial but similar advice may be offered to first-degree family members.

Key references

Balaji S. Long QT syndrome in children: not one disease anymore. *J Am Coll Cardiol* 2007;**50**:1341–2.

Border WL, Benson DW. Sudden infant death syndrome and long QT syndrome: The zealots versus the naysayers. *Heart Rhythm* 2007;**4**:167–9.

Goldenberg I, Moss AJ. Long QT syndrome. *J Am Coll Cardiol* 2008;**51**:2291–300.

Goldenberg I, Moss AJ, Zareba W. QT interval: how to measure it and what is "normal." *J Cardiovasc Electrophysiol* 2006;**17**:333–6.

Heidbüchel H, Corrado D, Biffi A, et al. Recommendations for participation in leisure-time physical activity and competitive sports of patients with arrhythmias and potentially arrhythmogenic conditions. Part II: ventricular arrhythmias, channelopathies and implantable defibrillators. *Eur J Cardiovasc Prev Rehabil* 2006;**13**:676–86.

Lupoglazoff JM, Denjoy I, Villain E, et al. Long QT syndrome in neonates: conduction disorders associated with HERG mutations and sinus bradycardia with KCNQ1 mutations. *J Am Coll Cardiol* 2004;**43**:826–30.

Maron BJ, Chaitman BR, Ackerman MJ, et al. Recommendations for physical activity and recreational sports participation for young patients with genetic cardiovascular diseases. *Circulation* 2004;**109**:2807–16.

Roden DM. Drug-induced prolongation of the QT interval. *N Engl J Med* 2004;**350**:1013–22.

Roden DM. Long-QT syndrome. *N Engl J Med* 2008;**358**:169–76.

Schwartz PJ, Moss AJ, Vincent GM, et al. Diagnostic criteria for the long QT syndrome: an update. *Circulation* 1993;**88**:782–4.

Schwartz PJ, Priori SG, Spazzolini C, et al. Genotype-phenotype correlation in the long-QT syndrome. *Circulation*. 2001;**103**:89–95.

Schwartz PJ, Spazzolini C, Crotti L, et al. The Jervell and Lange-Nielsen syndrome: natural history, molecular basis, and clinical outcome. *Circulation* 2006;**113**:783–90.

Schwartz PJ, Spazzolini C, Crotti L. All LQT3 patients need an ICD: true or false? *Heart Rhythm* 2008;**6**:113–20.

Schwartz PJ, Spazzolini C, Priori SG, et al. Who are the long-QT syndrome patients who receive an implantable cardioverter-defibrillator and what happens to them? *Circulation* 2010;**122**:1272–82.

Seth R, Moss AJ, McNitt S, et al. Long QT syndrome and pregnancy. *J Am Coll Cardiol* 2007;**49**:1092–8.

Vetter VL. Clues or miscues? How to make the right interpretation and correctly diagnose long-QT syndrome. *Circulation* 2007;**115**:2595–8.

Villain E, Denjoy I, Lupoglazoff JM, et al. Low incidence of cardiac events with beta-blocking therapy in children with long QT syndrome. *Eur Heart J* 2004;**25**:1405–11.

Vincent MG, Schwartz PJ, Denjoy I. High efficacy of β-blockers in long QT syndrome type 1: contribution of non-compliance and QT-prolonging drugs to the occurrence on treatment "failures". *Circulation* 2009;**119**:215–21.

www.fsm.it/cardmoc/

26 Catecholaminergic polymorphic ventricular tachycardia

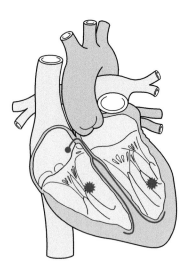

Catecholaminergic polymorphic ventricular tachycardia (CPVT) is one of the rarest but most dangerous ventricular arrhythmias encountered in childhood and is associated with a high risk of syncope and sudden death. It usually has autosomal dominant inheritance and 20–50% of cases show a mutation in the cardiac ryanodine receptor gene (*RYR2*). *RYR2* is the main calcium release channel on the sarcoplasmic reticulum within cardiac myocytes. Patients with an *RYR2* mutation are more likely to present in childhood and to be male compared with those with non-genotyped CPVT. Mutations in the cardiac calsequestrin gene (*CASQ2*) are described in a rare autosomal recessive form of CPVT.

ECG diagnosis

The ECG at rest is normal and the diagnosis is made from recordings on exercise. The ECG during exercise testing, Holter monitoring, or isoproterenol (isoprenaline) infusion generally shows a characteristic progression from ventricular premature beats to bidirectional ventricular tachycardia (VT) and/or polymorphic VT. Atrial premature beats or runs of atrial tachycardia are frequently seen in these patients. CPVT is also a possible underlying diagnosis in children with idiopathic ventricular fibrillation.

The ECG in Figure 26.1 shows the bidirectional VT characteristic of CPVT, in which alternate beats have an opposite QRS axis. It was recorded in a 9-year-old girl some while after she was rescued after a collapse in a swimming pool.

Concise Guide to Pediatric Arrhythmias, First Edition. Christopher Wren.
© 2012 John Wiley & Sons, Ltd. Published 2012 by John Wiley & Sons, Ltd.

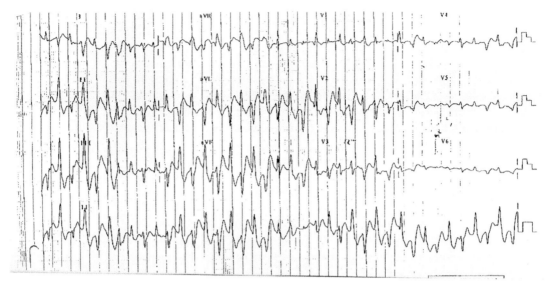

Figure 26.1

Figure 26.2 is a trace from a 7-year-old girl from a parent-activated event recorder immediately after a syncopal event in a swimming pool. It shows a few sinus beats followed by a run of bidirectional VT, which degenerates into faster polymorphic tachycardia and then returns to bidirectional VT. The patient survived and the diagnosis of CPVT was confirmed. Any history of syncope related to swimming strongly suggests either CPVT or long QT syndrome type 1.

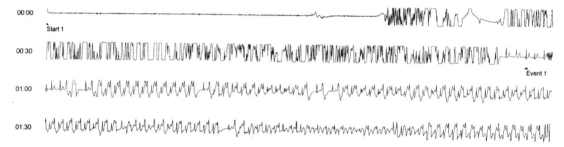

Figure 26.2

In the example in Figure 26.3 note that, even though alternate beats have different axes, the two axes are not constant, but change continually.

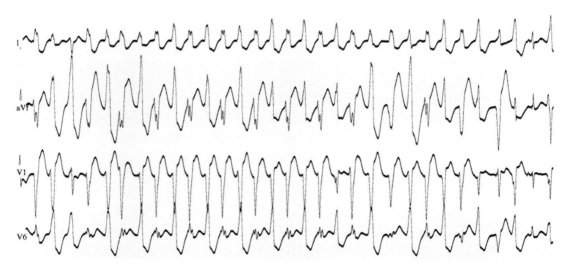

Figure 26.3

Treatment

Most reports suggest that β-blocker treatment gives a high degree of protection to patients with CPVT, but they are at great risk if the treatment is stopped or doses are missed. In older children and adolescents this risk will often be taken as an indication for an implantable defibrillator. The β-blocker of choice is nadolol, given at a dose of 1–2 mg/kg per day. The adequacy of the dose is confirmed by exercise or ambulatory ECG testing.

It seems that many children with CPVT have new mutations (10 of 14 [71%] in the report by Priori et al 2002). This is as one might expect because the natural history is to cause death before reproductive age. The implication of this finding is that the risk of siblings also having CPVT is probably more like 15% rather than 50%. In a report, Tester et al (2004) found *RYR2* mutations in 7 of 49 victims of sudden unexplained death with an age range of 2–34 years. This suggests that *RYR2* mutations might be a more common explanation for unexplained sudden cardiac death than has previously been realized.

Key references

Ackerman MJ, Tester DJ, Porter CJ. Swimming, a gene-specific arrhythmogenic trigger for inherited long QT syndrome. *Mayo Clin Proc* 1999;**74**:1088–94.

Choi G, Kopplin LJ, Tester DJ, et al. Spectrum and frequency of cardiac channel defects in swimming-triggered arrhythmia syndromes. *Circulation* 2004;**110**:2119–24.

Francis J, Sankar V, Krishnan Nair V, et al. Catecholaminergic polymorphic ventricular tachycardia. *Heart Rhythm* 2005;**2**:550–4.

Hayashi M, Denjoy I, Extramiana F, et al. Incidence and risk factors of arrhythmic events in catecholaminergic polymorphic ventricular tachycardia. *Circulation* 2009;**119**:2426–34.

Leenhardt A, Lucet V, Denjoy I, et al. Catecholaminergic polymorphic ventricular tachycardia in children. A 7-year follow-up of 21 patients. *Circulation* 1995;**91**:1512–19.

Napolitano C, Priori S. Diagnosis and treatment of catecholaminergic polymorphic ventricular tachycardia. *Heart Rhythm* 2007;**4**:675–8.

Priori SG, Napolitano C, Memmi M, et al. Clinical and molecular characterisation of patients with catecholaminergic polymorphic ventricular tachycardia. *Circulation* 2002;**106**:69–74.

Sumitomo N, Harada K, Nagashima M, et al. Catecholaminergic polymorphic ventricular tachycardia: electrocardiographic characteristics and optimal therapeutic strategies to prevent sudden death. *Heart* 2003;**89**:66–70.

Tester DJ, Spoon DB, Valdivia HH, et al. Targeted mutational analysis of the RyR2-endoded cardiac ryanodine receptor in sudden unexplained death: a molecular autopsy of 49 medical examiner/coroner's cases. *Mayo Clin Proc* 2004;**79**:1380–4.

27 Brugada syndrome

Brugada syndrome is a rare disease, mostly causing sudden death at rest from ventricular fibrillation in young men. It is rarely diagnosed in childhood although the original series did include three children. Brugada syndrome may come to light after investigation of syncope or cardiac arrest, or through investigation of a family history of sudden death. The differential diagnosis after presentation with ventricular fibrillation includes long QT syndrome, short QT syndrome, catecholaminergic polymorphic ventricular tachycardia, and idiopathic ventricular fibrillation as well as Brugada syndrome.

Brugada syndrome is dominantly inherited with very variable penetrance and in a minority of families is caused by a mutation of the *SCN5A* gene (other mutations of this gene are responsible for long QT syndrome type 3 – see Chapter 25). The genetic fault in most remains to be discovered.

Diagnosis

Brugada syndrome is characterized by downsloping ST elevation in right precordial leads on the ECG, which may be present at rest but is more often unmasked by intravenous administration of a sodium channel blocker, ajmaline or flecainide. The ECGs in Figures 27.1 and 27.2 are from an 11-year-old girl whose father died in his sleep at the age of 39 years. The autopsy was normal and the cause of his death was not established. His daughter's resting 12-lead ECG (Figure 27.1) showed an rSr′ pattern in lead V2 which could be a normal variant, but she showed a pattern of classic Brugada syndrome in response to administration of intravenous ajmaline (Figure 27.2). This response makes it likely that her father's death was as a result of Brugada syndrome.

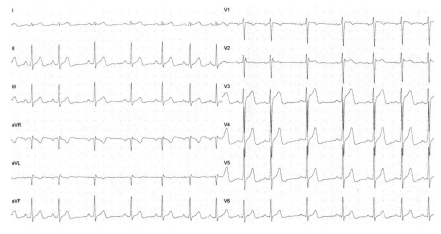

Figure 27.1

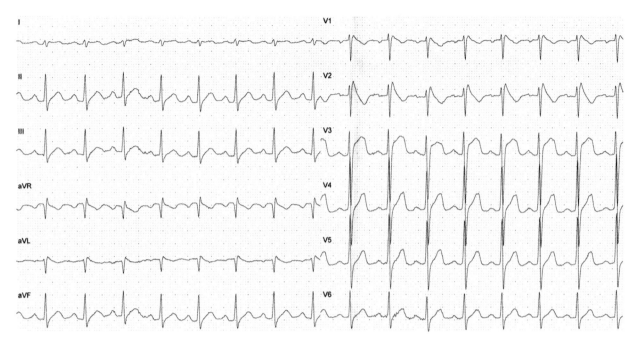

Figure 27.2

In the example in Figure 27.3, from a 15-year-old girl with a strong family history of Brugada syndrome, the response to a slow injection of flecainide 1 mg/kg can be seen. The ECG is normal at rest but within a few minutes develops downsloping ST elevation, most obvious in lead V2 (red arrow).

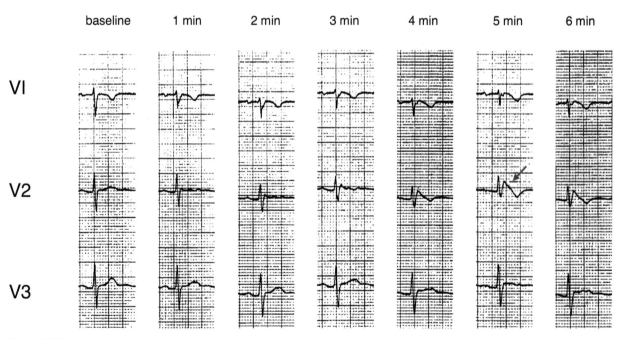

Figure 27.3

The population prevalence of the disease is unknown. A Brugada-like ECG may be present in up to $100/10^5$ adults. We have no estimate of the disease frequency in children but Japanese studies of children with an average age of 9 years found a Brugada-like ECG in $5–10/10^5$. A report of 30 children (only 11 of whom presented with syncope or cardiac arrest) with Brugada syndrome was compiled from 13 European centers – a measure of the disease rarity.

The risk of sudden death is higher in those with symptoms or with an abnormal ECG at baseline. A family history of sudden death appears not to be a risk factor and the risk is also lower if the ECG pattern of Brugada syndrome is apparent only after a drug challenge.

Treatment

It is often said that an implantable cardioverter/defibrillator (ICD) is the only effective therapy for Brugada syndrome but there is some recent evidence of benefit from treatment with quinidine.

There seems to be agreement that an ICD is indicated after resuscitation from ventricular fibrillation. It is less clear what should be done in asymptomatic patients with a normal resting ECG. The roles of pharmacological challenge and electrophysiology study with programmed stimulation are debated. The risk to asymptomatic children with affected family members seems to be very low so that it may be preferable to delay investigation until they are fully grown. The complications of an ICD in this population probably outweigh any benefit from treatment.

Syncope in children is often precipitated by fever so it is sometimes recommended that children should be admitted to hospital for observation and ECG monitoring if they develop a fever.

Key references

Brugada P, Brugada J. Right bundle branch block, persistent ST segment elevation and sudden cardiac death: a distinct clinical and electrocardiographic syndrome. A multicenter report. *J Am Coll Cardiol* 1992;**20**:1391–6.

Brugada P, Brugada R, Brugada J, Priori SG, Napolitano C. Should patients with an asymptomatic Brugada electrocardiogram undergo pharmacological and electrophysiological testing? *Circulation* 2005;**112**;279–92.

Probst V, Denjoy I, Meregalli PG, et al. Clinical aspects and prognosis of Brugada syndrome in children. *Circulation* 2007;**115**:2042–8.

Probst V, Veltmann C, Eckardt L, et al. Long-term prognosis of patients diagnosed with Brugada syndrome: Results from the FINGER Brugada Syndrome Registry. *Circulation* 2010;**121**:635–43.

Viskin S. Brugada syndrome in children. Don't ask, don't tell? *Circulation* 2007;**115**:1970–2.

Yamakawa Y, Ishikawa T, Uchino K, et al. Prevalence of right bundle branch block and right precordial ST-segment elevation (Brugada-type electrocardiogram) in Japanese children. *Circ J* 2004;**68**:275–9.

28 First- and second-degree atrioventricular block

First-degree atrioventricular block

First-degree atrioventricular (AV) block describes a prolonged PR interval on the ECG. It usually arises from delay in conduction through the AV node but a similar appearance may result from a delay in transatrial conduction – produced, for example, by drugs or Ebstein's anomaly. All P waves are conducted and first-degree block does not, in itself, cause bradycardia. The upper limit of a normal PR interval varies with age, from around 130 ms in infants to 170 ms in adults. First-degree block is often idiopathic and usually does not progress to more significant block during follow-up. It is also seen in atrioventricular septal defect, acute rheumatic fever, etc. The ECG in Figure 28.1 shows a PR interval of around 400 ms in a child with a small ventricular septal defect. AV conduction remained 1:1 during exercise testing and on ambulatory monitoring and did not change during 15 years of follow-up.

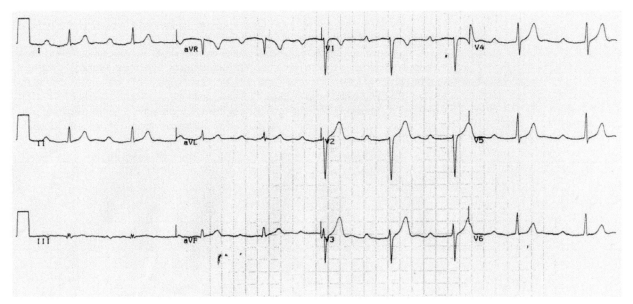

Figure 28.1

Second-degree atrioventricular block

In second-degree AV block some P waves are conducted and others are not. The type most commonly encountered is *Wenckebach block* (also known as Mobitz type I block) which is characterized by progressive lengthening of the PR interval

Concise Guide to Pediatric Arrhythmias, First Edition. Christopher Wren.
© 2012 John Wiley & Sons, Ltd. Published 2012 by John Wiley & Sons, Ltd.

before non-conduction of one beat. In the example in Figure 28.2, the PR interval lengthens over two or three beats before the third or fourth P wave is not conducted, so we have varying 3:2 and 4:3 conduction. P waves sometimes merge with the previous T waves and are less easy to see (arrows). In true Wenckebach conduction the PR interval increases by slightly less each beat so the RR interval shortens slightly and the longest RR is less than twice the shortest RR, as shown here.

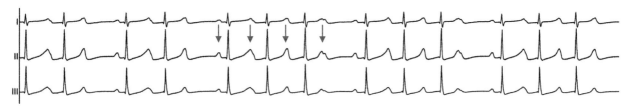

Figure 28.2

The example in Figure 28.3 first shows 3:2 Wenckebach conduction followed by 2:1 conduction. 2:1 AV conduction may result from Mobitz I or Mobitz II conduction but here it is clearly Mobitz I because of the 3:2 conduction.

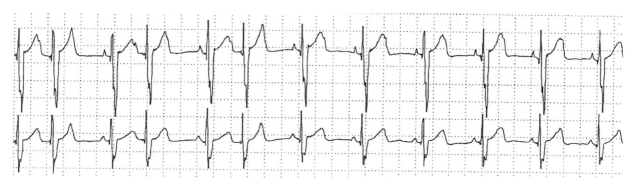

Figure 28.3

Wenckebach block is due to delay in conduction in the AV node. It is usually benign and does not require treatment. Transient nocturnal Wenckebach block is common in normal children.

Mobitz II block is very rare and implies an infranodal conduction delay. It is characterized by intermittent sudden failure of conduction in the absence of prolongation of the (normal) PR interval. Mobitz II block occurs in the presence of conduction system disease and there is almost always a wide QRS. It may be seen during recovery from early postoperative complete AV block. Mobitz II block is not benign and may be an indication for pacemaker implantation.

The rhythm strip in Figure 28.4 is from a 21-year-old man with congenitally corrected transposition of the great arteries. On ambulatory ECG recording he was noted to have non-conducted beats. This may not be classic Mobitz II block because he has a slightly prolonged PR interval all the time and his QRS is only slightly wider than normal. However, there is no preceding increase in the PR interval and the PR after the failure of conduction is the same as that before. The RR interval is double that in sinus rhythm. This is probably not an automatic indication for pacemaker implantation but in this clinical circumstance may be an indication for an electrophysiology study to investigate AV conduction.

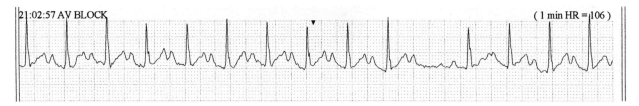

Figure 28.4

In the presence of stable 2:1, 3:1, or 4:1 conduction there is no opportunity to observe prolongation of the PR interval before the block, so characterization as Mobitz type I or type II AV block is not appropriate and this is best described as *high-grade second-degree AV block*. As shown in Figure 28.3, in 2:1 conduction a normal QRS complex and associated Wenckebach conduction show that AV nodal type I block is present, whereas a wide QRS complex may suggest the presence of infranodal type II block. Figure 28.5 shows stable 2:1 AV conduction in a neonate with a normal QRS. This is a rare finding and in this instance was associated with an aneurysm of the AV septum.

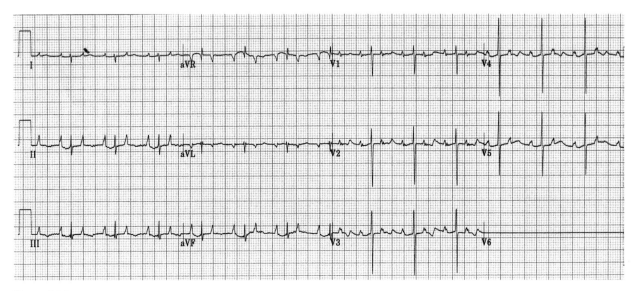

Figure 28.5

Figure 28.6 shows another example of constant 2:1 AV conduction from an asymptomatic teenager with a normal heart. This needs to be distinguished from non-conducted atrial bigeminy (see Chapter 11) but note that here the PP interval is regular and the P wave morphology is constant (this is best seen in more than one lead).

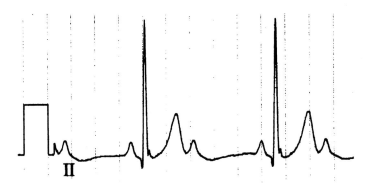

Figure 28.6

Key references

Mangrum JM, DiMarco JP. The evaluation and management of bradycardia. *N Engl J Med* 2000;**342**:703–9.

Scott O, Williams GJ, Fiddler GI. Results of 24 hour ambulatory monitoring of electrocardiogram in 131 healthy boys aged 10 to 13 years. *Br Heart J* 1980;**44**:304–8.

Sherron P, Torres-Arraut E, Tamer D, et al. Site of conduction delay and electrophysiologic significance of first-degree atrioventricular block in children with heart disease. *Am J Cardiol* 1985;**55**:1323–7.

Villain E, Bonnet D, Trigo C, et al. Outcome of, and risk factors for, second degree atrioventricular block in children. *Cardiol Young* 1996;**6**:315–19.

29 Complete atrioventricular block

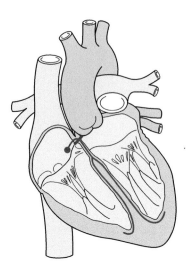

Complete atrioventricular (AV) block describes the absence of electrical conduction from the atria to the ventricles. The ECG shows P waves at an appropriate rate for age and a regular ventricular bradycardia with AV dissociation. The QRS may be normal or show changes related to underlying structural heart disease or previous surgery. Complete AV block may be an isolated abnormality, or related to structural cardiovascular malformations (such as left atrial isomerism or congenitally corrected transposition of the great arteries), or associated with myopathies (see Chapter 34), or caused by intracardiac repair of a cardiac malformation.

Etiology of isolated complete AV block

Isolated AV block in the fetus or newborn occurs in around 1 in 20 000 pregnancies. It is almost always related to the presence of Sjögren's syndrome antibodies (anti-Ro and anti-La antibodies) in the mother. Most of these women are asymptomatic but some have rheumatoid arthritis, systemic lupus erythematosus, Sjögren's syndrome, or other connective tissue disease. An antibody-positive woman has a risk of producing a baby with complete AV block of around 2%, with a recurrence risk of 15% for subsequent offspring if AV block does occur. The precise pathophysiology is not well understood. Mothers of infants older than 28 days at diagnosis or children with newly recognized AV block are usually antibody negative, and the cause is then unknown.

ECG diagnosis of complete AV block

Complete AV block is easily recognized from the ECG. P waves occur at a normal rate for age with no evidence of AV conduction. This means that the ventricular bradycardia is *regular*. In the newborn baby the QRS is usually normal, as in Figure 29.1. In this example the atrial rate is 142/min and the ventricular rate 68/min. P waves are easily seen (red arrows) and the QRS complexes are regular.

Concise Guide to Pediatric Arrhythmias, First Edition. Christopher Wren.
© 2012 John Wiley & Sons, Ltd. Published 2012 by John Wiley & Sons, Ltd.

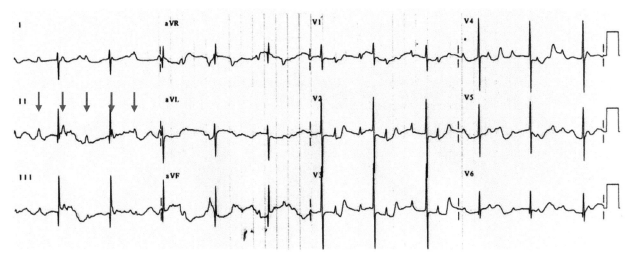

Figure 29.1

Sometimes, as shown in Figure 29.2, the ventricular rate is almost exactly half the atrial rate and a longer recording may be necessary to confirm complete dissociation and to rule out 2:1 AV conduction or sinus bradycardia.

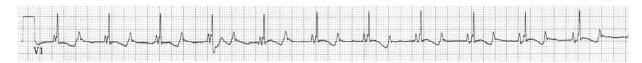

Figure 29.2

The ventricular rate varies greatly between patients and can also respond significantly to exercise. Figure 29.3 shows a rhythm strip from a neonate with a ventricular rate of around 75/min. The diagnosis had been made prenatally, when the ventricular rate was around 95.min.

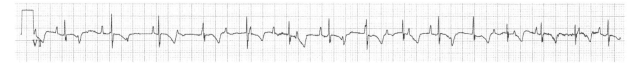

Figure 29.3

The ventricular rate tends to slow with age and all patients will eventually require pacemaker implantation. Figure 29.4, from the same child as in Figure 29.3, shows that the ventricular rate has fallen to 65/min by the age of 2 years.

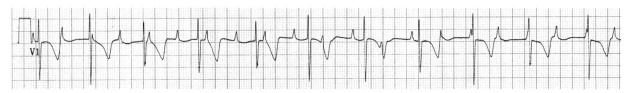

Figure 29.4

The ECG in Figure 29.5 is from a 12-year-old girl who presented with syncope. The ventricular bradycardia is profound, with a rate of 28/min. Her heart was structurally normal and the poor R wave progression in the chest leads probably reflects ventricular dilation. The age of onset of her heart block, and its cause, remain unknown. However, an ECG in the referring hospital records, when she was seen with a murmur at 4 years of age, also showed complete AV block (which had not been recognized), and bradycardia had been recorded when she had a tonsillectomy age 7, and when she was admitted with gastroenteritis aged 1 year.

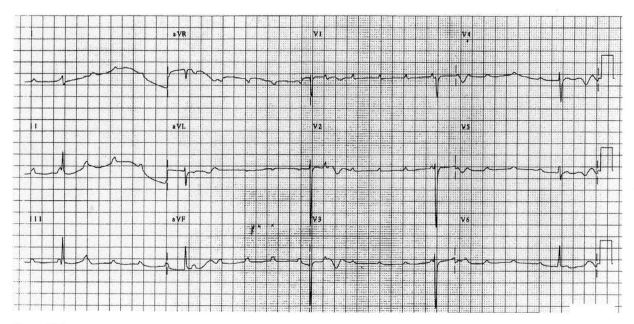

Figure 29.5

If complete AV block is seen in postoperative patients, or occurs in association with structural congenital heart disease, the QRS is likely to be abnormal. In the ECG in Figure 29.6 the underlying diagnosis is congenitally corrected transposition of the great arteries (atrioventricular and ventriculo-arterial discordance). Note the QRS axis of around +20° with deep Q waves in lead V1 and absence of Q waves in lead V6.

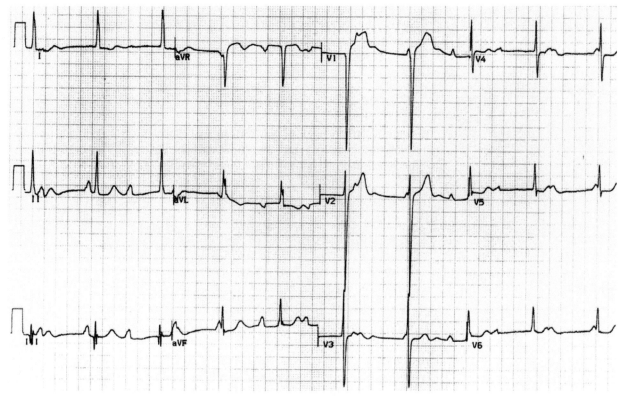

Figure 29.6

Indications for pacing

Most or all children with AV block will require permanent pacemaker implantation before reaching adulthood, probably more than half of them in the first year of life. Pacing is generally thought to be indicated in neonates who have signs of heart failure (which is unusual) or a persisting bradycardia <55/min. The recording in Figure 29.7 is from a neonate and the ventricular rate of 48/min, coupled with breathlessness and signs of heart failure, was taken as an indication for pacemaker implantation.

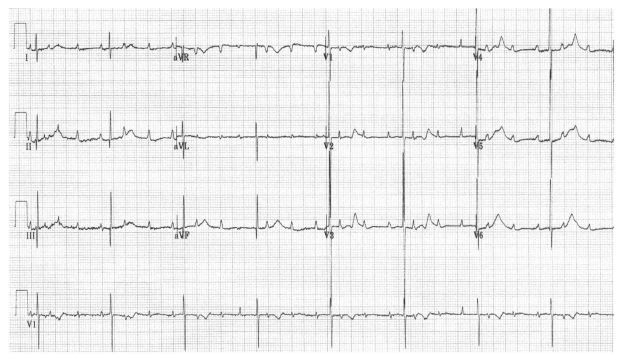

Figure 29.7

In children the main indication is a persisting *daytime* ventricular rate <50/min, especially if this is accompanied by sudden pauses in the escape rhythm or failure of the ventricular rate to track a rise in atrial rate with exercise. By the early teens more or less all children with complete AV block will have received a pacemaker. It is noteworthy that most remain asymptomatic and syncope or presyncope is an unusual indication for pacing. However, older children undergoing pacing for the first time do report an improvement in wellbeing and exercise ability, even though they considered themselves to be completely well before pacing.

The lower limit of acceptable ventricular rate is higher in the presence of structural congenital heart disease although the limit is not defined. Figure 29.8 shows an ECG recorded many years ago from an asymptomatic 5-year-old boy with congenitally corrected transposition of the great arteries. The ventricular rate is <40/min and should have been an indication for pacemaker implantation. Sadly that was not done and he died suddenly several weeks after this ECG was recorded.

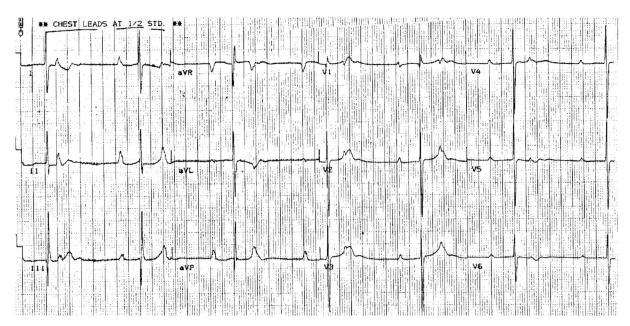

Figure 29.8

Postoperative complete AV block that persists for more than 10 days after surgery is an absolute indication for pacemaker implantation. Recovery of normal AV conduction after this time is rare. The ECG in Figure 29.9 was recorded in an 18-month-old girl after resection of recurrent severe fibromuscular subaortic stenosis. It shows a ventricular rate of around 75/min with a wide QRS escape rhythm. She received a permanent pacemaker. Pacemaker implantation is discussed in Chapter 38.

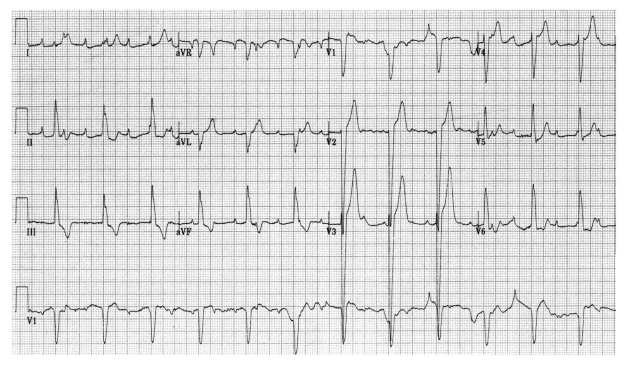

Figure 29.9

Key references

Balmer C, Fasnacht M, Rahn M, et al. Long-term follow up of children with congenital complete atrioventricular block and the impact of pacemaker therapy. *Europace* 2002;**4**:345–9.

Dewey RC, Capeless MA, Levy AM. Use of ambulatory electrocardiographic monitoring to identify high-risk patients with congenital complete heart block. *N Engl J Med* 1987;**316**:835–9.

Epstein AE, DiMarco JP, Ellenbogen KA, et al. ACC/AHA/HRS 2008 Guidelines for device-based therapy of cardiac rhythm abnormalities: a report of the American College of Cardiology/American Heart Association Task Force on Practice Guidelines. *Circulation* 2008;**117**:e350–408.

Eronen M, Siren MK, Ekblad H, et al. Short- and long-term outcome of children with congenital complete heart block diagnosed *in utero* or as a newborn. *Pediatrics* 2000;**106**:86–91.

Friedman RA. Congenital AV block. Pace me now or pace me later? *Circulation* 1995;**92**:283–5.

Gross GJ, Chiu CC, Hamilton RM, et al. Natural history of postoperative heart block in congenital heart disease: implications for pacing intervention. *Heart Rhythm* 2006;**3**:601–4.

Jaeggi ET, Hamilton RM, Silverman ED, et al. Outcome of children with fetal, neonatal or childhood diagnosis of isolated congenital atrioventricular block A single institution's experience of 30 years. *J Am Coll Cardiol* 2002;**39**:130–7.

Michaëlsson M, Jonzon A, Riesenfeld T. Isolated congenital complete atrioventricular block in adult life. A prospective study. *Circulation* 1995;**92**:283–5.

Michaelsson M, Riesenfeld T, Jonzon A. Natural history of congenital complete atrioventricular block. *Pacing Clin Electrophysiol* 1997;**20**:2098–101.

Villain E. Indications for pacing in patients with congenital heart disease. *Pacing Clin Electrophysiol* 2008;**31**(suppl 1):S17–20.

Villain E, Coastedoat-Chalumeau N, Marijon E, et al. Presentation and prognosis of complete atrioventricular block in childhood, according to maternal antibody status. *J Am Coll Cardiol* 2006;**48**:1682–7.

Weindling SN, Saul JP, Gamble WJ, et al. Duration of complete atrioventricular block after congenital heart disease surgery. *Am J Cardiol* 1998;**82**:525–7.

30 Sinus node dysfunction and sinoatrial disease

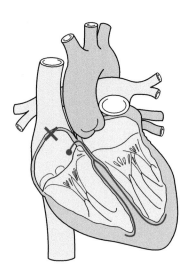

Symptomatic sinus node dysfunction is rare in children with structurally normal hearts and very little has been written about it in recent years. It may occur in association with structural heart disease or after surgical repair of cardiac defects.

Sinus node dysfunction describes abnormalities of sinus node automaticity and sinoatrial conduction that produce a variety of ECG abnormalities, including sinus bradycardia, sinus pauses, sinus arrest, sinoatrial block, and atrial tachycardias.

Sinoatrial disease (also known as sinuatrial disease and sick sinus syndrome) describes the clinical combination of symptoms and ECG evidence of sinus node dysfunction. The disease process is not confined to the sinus node as atrial arrhythmias and atrioventricular (AV) conduction abnormalities are sometimes seen. Sinoatrial disease with atrial arrhythmias is sometimes known as bradycardia–tachycardia syndrome.

Abnormal sinus node function is sometimes observed as a secondary phenomenon. In preterm neonates it is common in response to apnea. In infants and young children prolonged sinus arrest with absence of any escape rhythm is seen in reflex asystolic syncope. In older children it may be a manifestation of increased vagal tone, sometimes associated with syncope.

Sinoatrial disease is rare in children. Most of the cases reported are in boys and it sometimes occurs as a familial disease. The main symptoms reported are dizziness, presyncope, and syncope. ECG abnormalities may be apparent at rest or may be correlated with symptoms during ambulatory ECG recording.

Figure 30.1 shows non-consecutive rhythm strips from an ambulatory ECG recording from a 14-year-old boy with a history of palpitations and dizziness. They show pauses due to both absence of and failure to conduct P waves. There is intermittent atrial tachycardia and more than one P wave shape.

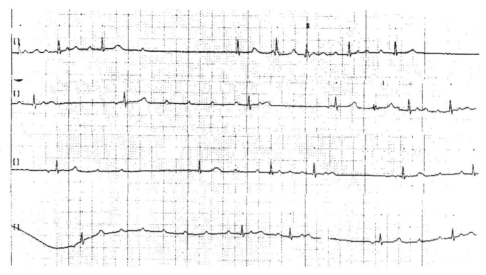

Figure 30.1

Further non-consecutive recordings in Figure 30.2 from the same boy show episodes of atrial tachycardia with 1:1 AV conduction. The QRS complexes sometimes show rate-related aberration

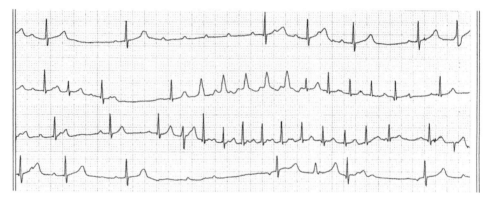

Figure 30.2

The ECG in Figure 30.3, from an asymptomatic infant, shows a junctional escape rhythm with occasional P waves just behind or just ahead of the QRS (arrows).

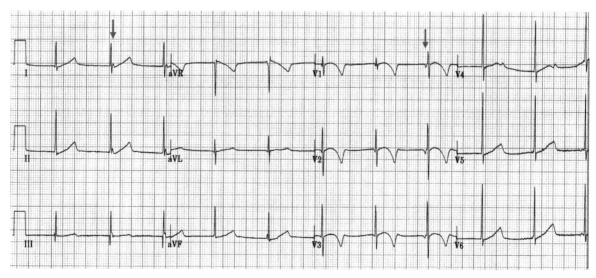

Figure 30.3

Sinus node dysfunction is common after operations involving suture lines close to the sinus node, notably atrial baffle repairs of transposition of the great arteries and repair of sinus venosus atrial septal defect (see Chapter 32). The example in Figure 30.4 is from a Holter recording in an asymptomatic 20-year-old man who had undergone a Senning operation in infancy. It shows a sudden slowing of sinus rhythm followed by sinus bradycardia.

+07:47:06 Brady HR = 27 bpm   (1 min HR = 32)

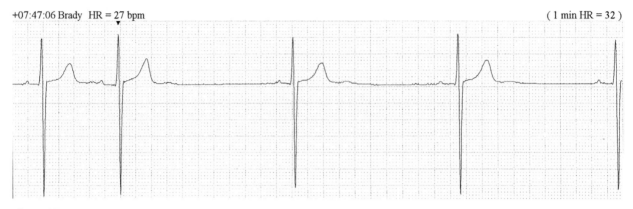

Figure 30.4

Treatment

Decisions about treatment depend on the presence or absence of symptoms and on the clinical situation. It is rare to recommend treatment of asymptomatic ECG abnormalities. Chronic arrhythmias with symptoms may require treatment. Pacemaker implantation is the definitive treatment if warranted by symptoms. Atrial pacing may be sufficient if AV conduction is normal but ventricular pacing or dual chamber pacing is more often employed, particularly as the patient is likely to be most often in sinus rhythm. Atrial tachycardias may be treated with a β-blocker or digoxin, or sometimes with other antiarrhythmic drugs, but this may exacerbate bradycardia and necessitate pacemaker implantation.

Key references

Benson DW, Wang DW, Dyment M. Congenital sick sinus syndrome caused by recessive mutations in the cardiac sodium channel gene (SCN5A). *J Clin Invest* 2003;**112**:1019–28.

Friedli B. Sino-atrial disease. In Wren C, Campbell RWF (eds). *Paediatric cardiac arrhythmias*. 1996. Oxford University Press.

Kugler JD. Sinus node dysfunction. *Prog Pediatr Cardiol* 1994;**3**:226–35.

Mackintosh AF. Sinuatrial disease in young people. *Br Heart J* 1981;**45**:62–6.

Mangrum JM, DiMarco JP. The evaluation and management of bradycardia. *N Engl J Med* 2000;**342**:703–9.

Park DS, Fishman GI. The cardiac conduction system. *Circulation* 2011;**123**:904–15.

Yabek SM, Dillon T, Berman W Jr, et al. Symptomatic sinus node dysfunction in children without structural heart disease. *Pediatrics* 1982;**69**:590–3.

Early postoperative arrhythmias

Hemodynamically significant arrhythmias are frequent in the early days after pediatric cardiac surgery, affecting perhaps 15–20% of cases overall. They are more common after open than after closed operations, in smaller patients, and in those who have undergone more complex intracardiac repair. Diagnosis and management are made easier by routine placement of temporary epicardial atrial and ventricular pacing wires. Any arrhythmia may be seen but those discussed below are the most important.

Tachycardias

Sinus tachycardia is very common after surgery and may be caused by pain, fever, infusion of inotropic drugs, etc. Although it is usually not considered to be an arrhythmia, it sometimes needs to be distinguished from more significant arrhythmias, particularly junctional ectopic tachycardia. Administration of adenosine will usually cause gradual slowing of sinus tachycardia followed by acceleration as the effect of the drug wears off, as seen in Figure 31.1.

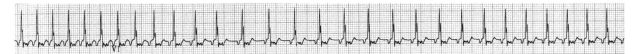

Figure 31.1

Sometimes adenosine will slow sinus tachycardia and then suppress atrial activity transiently so that there is a nodal or junctional rhythm for a few seconds, as shown in Figure 31.2.

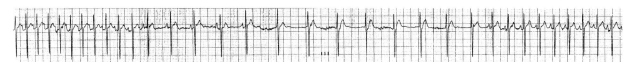

Figure 31.2

Occasionally postoperative sinus tachycardia can cause hemodynamic problems. This is most likely when there is also first-degree atrioventricular (AV) block, causing the P wave to occur in the previous ST segment. As a result the atria contract during ventricular systole and cardiac output is reduced. In the example in Figure 31.3, P waves cannot be seen in the rhythm strip (upper panel) but are easily identified with an atrial electrogram (red arrow, middle panel). The diagnosis is confirmed

Concise Guide to Pediatric Arrhythmias, First Edition. Christopher Wren.
© 2012 John Wiley & Sons, Ltd. Published 2012 by John Wiley & Sons, Ltd.

by adenosine administration which causes sinus slowing and transient junctional rhythm (middle panel) – contrast this with junctional ectopic tachycardia below. The solution is to use temporary AV pacing with a short AV interval (bottom panel).

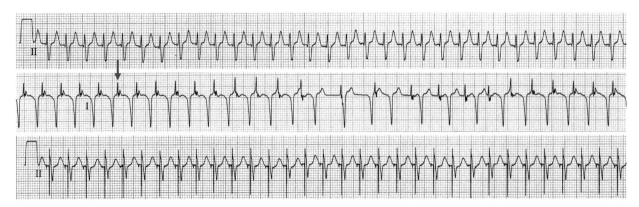

Figure 31.3

Junctional ectopic tachycardia is the most significant early postoperative tachycardia, usually developing a few hours after return to the intensive care unit. It is characterized by atrial dissociation, as discussed below. It originates close to the His bundle and is caused by hemorrhage or edema in tissues around the AV junction. It most often affects infants who have had intracardiac repair of malformations such as tetralogy of Fallot, ventricular septal defect, or atrioventricular septal defect. At lower ventricular rates, the diagnosis is straightforward, with regular QRS complexes and slower dissociated P waves, as seen Figure 31.4 (black arrows). There may be occasional sinus capture beats which make the QRS complexes slightly irregular (red arrows – see also chapter 17). The QRS complexes are usually normal in morphology but may show a right bundle branch block (RBBB) pattern after an operation such as repair of tetralogy of Fallot or a left bundle branch block (LBBB) pattern after surgery on the left ventricular outflow.

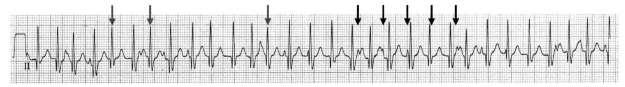

Figure 31.4

If P waves are not easy to see on the surface ECG, it is helpful to record an atrial electrogram from temporary epicardial pacing wires. Atrial electrical activity will then be revealed and slower dissociated P waves will confirm the diagnosis, as shown in Figure 31.5 (red arrows).

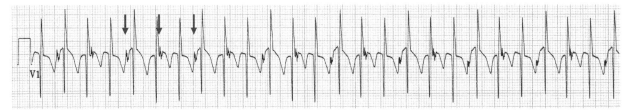

Figure 31.5

Sometimes junctional ectopic tachycardia exhibits 1:1 retrograde ventriculoatrial (VA) conduction, making diagnosis more difficult. The solution is to give intravenous adenosine which will cause temporary retrograde block and produce VA dissociation, confirming the diagnosis. In the example in Figure 31.6 the rhythm is at first regular with no visible P waves. Adenosine then produces retrograde block and dissociated P waves are visible at a rate slightly slower than the QRS complexes (arrows).

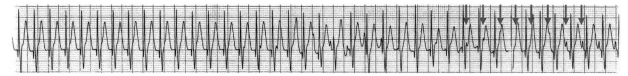

Figure 31.6

Junctional ectopic tachycardia can be a very significant problem in the short term, contributing to hemodynamic compromise. It does not respond to DC cardioversion and cannot be terminated by overdrive pacing. Any underlying metabolic or biochemical abnormality should be corrected and patients weaned off doses of inotropic drugs if possible. Active management usually involves a combination of cooling to around 34–35 °C, amiodarone infusion, and pacing. The aim of treatment is usually rate control rather than necessarily maintaining sinus rhythm. Overdrive atrial pacing will restore AV synchrony at the expense of a slightly higher ventricular rate. AV synchrony can also be provided by using VA sequential pacing to overcome VA block, and to position the P wave in front of the following QRS. This is achieved by reversing the atrial and ventricular leads but can be difficult to set up and maintain. Early postoperative junctional ectopic tachycardia is usually only a short-term problem and most often runs its course within 3–5 days, after which treatment can be withdrawn.

Atrial tachycardia and atrial flutter

A variety of atrial arrhythmias may be seen early after cardiac surgery. Some will affect infants or children with previous arrhythmias but more commonly the arrhythmia is new. Most atrial tachycardias occur at a high enough rate for there to be AV block (most commonly 2:1) but this is not always easy to see on the surface ECG. Diagnosis is helped either by recording an ECG from epicardial atrial wires or by giving adenosine. In the example in Figure 31.7, from a 9-year-old girl who had undergone a tricuspid valve replacement, there is an irregular tachycardia but it is not easy to make out P waves on the surface ECG. In Figure 31.8 the left and right arm leads are connected to the temporary atrial electrodes. This means that lead I produces an atrial electrogram and other leads show hybrid recordings with superimposed atrial electrograms. It is easy to see that there is a regular atrial tachycardia at about 300/min (arrows) with variable AV conduction.

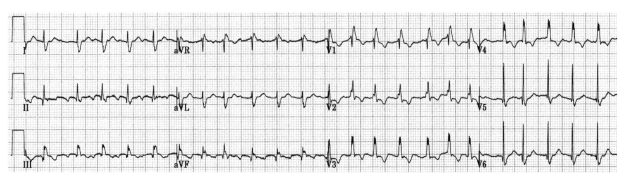

Figure 31.7

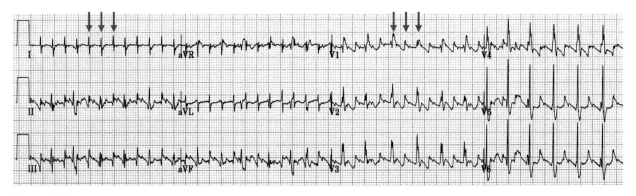

Figure 31.8

In Figure 31.9, from a teenager who underwent AV valve repair in a failing Fontan circulation, the rhythm is irregular and is not obviously sinus but is difficult to make out.

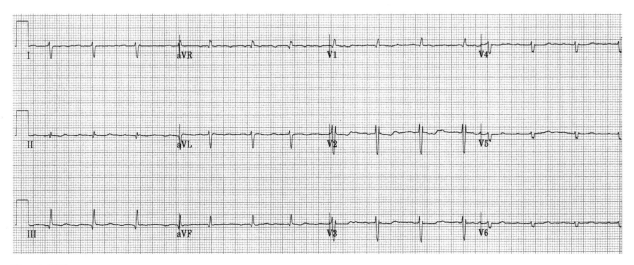

Figure 31.9

By attaching lead V1 to a temporary epicardial atrial wire (Figure 31.10), the rhythm becomes clear. There is an atrial tachycardia at around 250/min with variable AV conduction. The sharp deflections represent P waves and the smaller deflections are QRS complexes (red arrows).

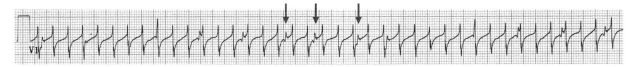

Figure 31.10

In another example in Figure 31.11 the rhythm is difficult to make out on the surface ECG, but is obviously not sinus, with low amplitude electrical activity and regular QRS complexes.

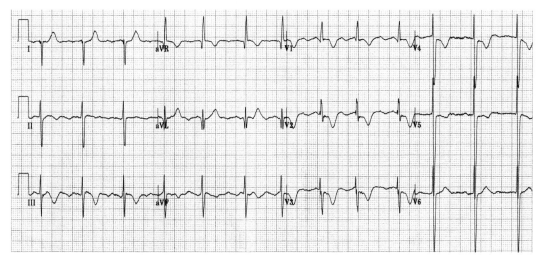

Figure 31.11

The situation is made clearer by recording an atrial electrogram (Figure 31.12). There is an atrial tachycardia at around 280/min but notice also that there is AV dissociation caused by complete AV block.

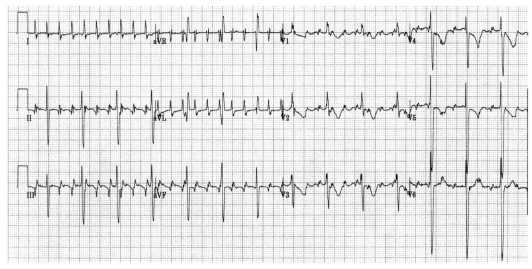

Figure 31.12

The recording in Figure 31.13 is from a 3-year-old boy who developed a sustained tachycardia after atrial baffle revision (having previously had a double-switch operation for congenitally corrected transposition of the great arteries). The diagnosis becomes clear with adenosine administration, which produces temporary AV block and unmasks atrial flutter.

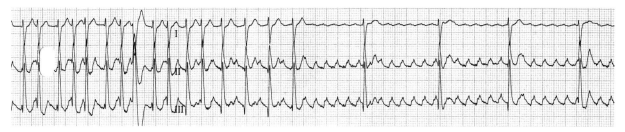

Figure 31.13

The management of early postoperative atrial tachycardia depends on the clinical situation. Usually the priority will be to restore sinus rhythm by overdrive atrial pacing or DC cardioversion. If this is the first episode of arrhythmia and the underlying cardiac function is good, it may not be necessary to start drug treatment. If there have been previous episodes of cardiac arrhythmia and there are residual hemodynamic abnormalities, it may be beneficial to reduce the risk of a recurrence by giving amiodarone or a β-blocker.

Atrioventricular re-entry tachycardia is a common arrhythmia in children with a normal heart but may also occur in those with structural heart disease and is sometimes seen for the first time early after surgery. Diagnosis is usually straightforward; there is 1:1 AV conduction and tachycardia can be stopped with intravenous adenosine or overdrive pacing. Prophylactic antiarrhythmic medication is not necessarily indicated if there has been no preoperative occurrence of arrhythmia (see Chapter 12).

Early postoperative *atrial ectopic tachycardia* is a rare arrhythmia but is reported (see Chapter 7). It is most often seen after repair of transposition of the great arteries with previous atrial septostomy. It usually occurs as a single episode. Sometimes it is well tolerated and does not require treatment, resolving spontaneously within a few days. If necessary, treatment involves correction of hypokalemia, reduction in inotrope infusions, and oral or intravenous β-blocker therapy.

Atrial fibrillation is a very rare pediatric arrhythmia but may be seen after surgery in older teenagers and young adults (see Chapter 10). If it is a new arrhythmia it most commonly resolves within 24 hours so treatment may not be necessary. Rate control can be achieved with calcium channel blockers, β-blocking agents, digoxin, or amiodarone. It is important also to correct factors such as pain, hemodynamic instability, weaning of intravenous inotropes, electrolyte and metabolic abnormalities, anemia, or hypoxia. DC cardioversion may be indicated if there is hemodynamic instability or the arrhythmia persists beyond 24 hours. If recurrence is thought likely, consideration should be given to prophylaxis with metoprolol, sotalol, amiodarone, or other antiarrhythmic drugs. Warfarin may be indicated to reduce the risk of stroke.

Early postoperative *atrial premature beats* are common and usually benign, requiring no treatment (see Chapter 11). Occasionally they may cause hemodynamic disturbance. In the example in Figure 31.14, from a neonate with repaired total anomalous pulmonary venous connection, there are frequent atrial premature beats, some of which are conducted (black arrows) and some of which are blocked (red arrows), producing alternating bradycardia and tachycardia. This arrhythmia proved unresponsive to amiodarone but resolved quickly after administration of oral propranolol.

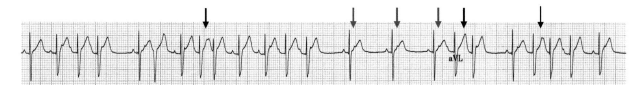

Figure 31.14

Ventricular premature beats are common but usually cause no haemodynamic disturbance and require no treatment (see Chapter 23). If necessary, any treatable cause should be investigated as discussed below for ventricular tachycardia.

Early postoperative *ventricular tachycardia* is uncommon (see Chapter 18). When it does occur it is usually non-sustained and often related to myocardial disease, ischemia, or dysfunction. In these situations the QRS complexes may be broad and bizarre. As with several other early postoperative arrhythmias, every effort should be made to correct any contributing factors such as electrolyte imbalances, metabolic acidosis, and intracardiac pressure lines that may have migrated to a ventricle. It is difficult to generalize about treatment. If emergency treatment is required because of loss of cardiac output, give a synchronized DC shock of 0.5–1 J/kg, followed by 2 J/kg if the first is ineffective. If there is more time to respond, intravenous calcium or magnesium may stabilize the situation. Magnesium sulfate 25–50 mg/kg (0.1–0.2 mmol/kg) is given over 10–15 min and repeated once if necessary. The maximum dose is 2 g.

If antiarrhythmic drug treatment is thought necessary, the choice is between amiodarone and lidocaine (usually in a dose of 1 mg/kg followed by an infusion of 20–50 μg/kg per min). Intravenous esmolol may also be useful on occasion. The rhythm strip in Figure 31.15 is from a 5-year-old girl who had respiratory arrest after replacement of a right ventricular outflow conduit and developed secondary myocardial ischemia. It shows a regular wide QRS tachycardia of 240/min. Ventricular tachycardia was proven by dissociated P waves on the 12-lead ECG (not easy to see here) but in this situation atrial dissociation could also be demonstrated by an atrial electrogram or a right atrial pressure trace.

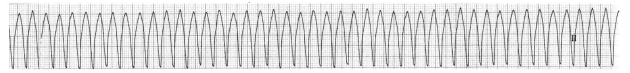

Figure 31.15

Ventricular fibrillation is not uncommon as an intraoperative or immediate postoperative arrhythmia – perhaps occurring in up to 1% of cases. It is usually related to myocardial ischemia, because of either an intrinsic coronary artery abnormality or poor myocardial perfusion, particularly if there is also previously impaired ventricular function. Thus, it may occur after an arterial switch for transposition of the great arteries, repair of anomalous origin of the left coronary artery from the pulmonary artery, or a Norwood operation. Other possible contributing causes include coronary air embolism, and inadvertent overadministration of drugs, intravenous potassium replacements, etc.

If ventricular fibrillation occurs, cardiopulmonary resuscitation should be started immediately. An unsynchronized shock of 2 J/kg is given as soon as possible. Resuscitation is continued and, if a reasonable rhythm with good cardiac output is not restored immediately, a second shock of 4 J/kg is given. If this does not work, intravenous epinephrine 0.01 mg/kg (0.1 mL/kg 1:10 000) is given. Chest compressions are continued and the DC shock and epinephrine repeated as necessary. If ventricular fibrillation continues, amiodarone 5 mg/kg or lidocaine 1 mg/kg is given. If defibrillation is successful but ventricular fibrillation recurs, chest compression is continued, another bolus of amiodarone given, and then an attempt to defibrillate with the previously successful DC shock dose is made. Once sinus rhythm, or other rhythm with cardiac output, is restored, the underlying cause of ventricular fibrillation should be searched for and corrected.

Bradycardias

Sinus bradycardia is common and easily overcome by atrial pacing at an appropriate rate to optimize the cardiac output. It is usually transient and is rarely an indication for permanent pacing.

Sinus node dysfunction is most often seen after operations involving suture lines close to the sinus node or its blood supply. These include repair of sinus venosus atrial septal defect, hemi-Fontan operation, lateral tunnel total cavopulmonary connection, and a Senning operation or other atrial baffle operations. The definition of sinus node dysfunction varies in different reports. However, it is usually recognized in this situation by either the absence of normal sinus P waves with a slow atrial or junctional rhythm, or the presence of sinus pauses. Sinus node dysfunction can be overcome in the short term by temporary atrial pacing and will usually resolve or improve spontaneously with time. There may occasionally be an indication for late pacemaker implantation.

Postoperative *complete AV block* was common in an earlier era, when less was known about the anatomy of the conduction tissue in complex malformations. Surgeons now have a detailed knowledge of the course of the AV node and bundle of His in all including the most complex malformations. However, AV block still occurs, with a higher risk in smaller infants undergoing complex intracardiac repair.

AV block is usually transient and managed by temporary epicardial pacing at an appropriate rate. If spontaneous return of sinus rhythm were to occur it would nearly always do so within 10 days. If AV block persists for longer than this, it is highly probable that a permanent pacemaker will be required.

The ECG in Figure 31.16 is from an 18-month-old girl after resection of recurrent severe fibromuscular subaortic stenosis. The atrial rate is about 160/min (red arrows) and there is a regular ventricular bradycardia with a rate of 75/min with complete AV dissociation. The QRS complexes are wide with an appearance similar to LBBB. AV conduction did not recover and a permanent pacemaker was implanted before discharge from hospital.

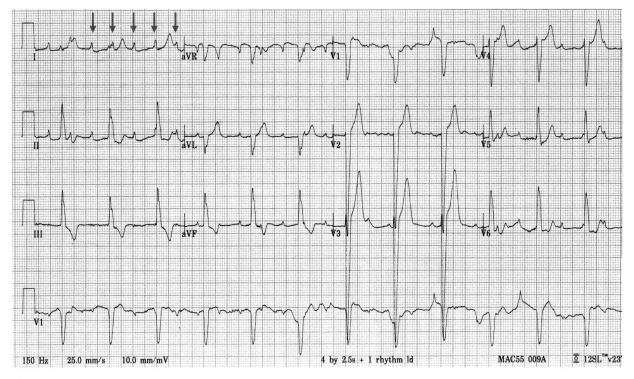

Figure 31.16

In the ECG in Figure 31.17, from a 5 year old after AV valve replacement in a Fontan circulation, the atrial rate is 115/min and the ventricular rate 90/min. In the top trace, lead aVF, the P waves (red arrows) are larger than the QRS complexes. The AV block resolved and pacing was not required.

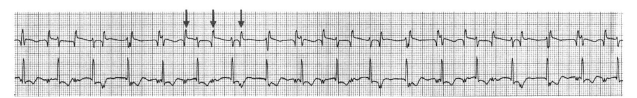

Figure 31.17

Temporary epicardial pacing may also be used in the absence of AV block to optimize cardiac output by improving ventricular synchrony. This can be achieved by adjusting the AV interval and/or using multisite ventricular pacing, usually to improve the function of a subpulmonary right ventricle.

Key references

Delaney JW, Moltedo JM, Dziura JD, et al. Early postoperative arrhythmias after pediatric cardiac surgery. *J Thorac Cardiovasc Surg* 2006;**131**:1296–300.

Drew BJ, Califf RM, Funk M, et al. Practice standards for electrocardiographic monitoring in hospital settings. *Circulation* 2004;**110**:2721–46.

Haas NA, Camphausen CK. Impact of early and standardized treatment with amiodarone on therapeutic success and outcome in pediatric patients with postoperative tachyarrhythmia. *J Thorac Cardiovasc Surg* 2008;**136**:1215–22.

Janousek J. Cardiac resynchronisation in congenital heart disease. *Heart* 2009;**95**:940–7.

Kleinman ME, Chameides L, Schexnayder SM, et al. Pediatric Advanced Life Support: 2010 American Heart Association guidelines for cardiopulmonary resuscitation and emergency cardiovascular care. *Circulation* 2010;**122**:S876–908.

Kovacikova L, Hakacova N, Dobos D, et al. Amiodarone as a first-line therapy for postoperative junctional ectopic tachycardia. *Ann Thorac Surg* 2009;**88**:616–22.

Manrique AM, Arroyo M, Lin Y, et al. Magnesium supplementation during cardiopulmonary bypass to prevent junctional ectopic tachycardia after pediatric cardiac surgery: A randomized controlled study. *J Thorac Cardiovasc Surg* 2010;**139**:162–9.

Moltedo JM, Rosenthal GL, Delaney J, et al. The utility and safety of temporary pacing wires in postoperative patients with congenital heart disease. *J Thorac Cardiovasc Surg* 2007;**134**:515–16.

Rho RW. The management of atrial fibrillation after cardiac surgery. *Heart* 2009;**95**:422–9.

Rosales AM, Walsh EP, Wessel DL, et al. Postoperative atrial tachycardia in children with congenital heart disease. *Am J Cardiol* 2001;**88**:1169–72.

Silva JNA, Van Hare GF. Management of postoperative pediatric cardiac arrhythmias: current state of the art. *Curr Treat Options Cardiovasc Med* 2009;**11**:410–16.

Valsangiacomo E, Schmid ER, Schüpbach RW, et al. Early postoperative arrhythmias after cardiac operation in children. *Ann Thorac Surg* 2002;**74**:792–6.

Van Hare GF. Ventricular fibrillation in the postoperative cardiac patient. In: Quan L, Franklin WH (eds), *Ventricular fibrillation: a pediatric problem*. Armonk, NY: Futura Publishing Co. Inc., 2000: 115–26.

Walsh EP, Saul JP, Sholler GF, et al. Evaluation of a staged treatment protocol for rapid automatic junctional tachycardia after operation for congenital heart disease. *J Am Coll Cardiol* 1997;**29**:1046–53.

Weindling SN, Saul JP, Gamble WJ, et al. Duration of complete atrioventricular block after congenital heart disease surgery. *Am J Cardiol* 1998;**82**:525–7.

32 Late postoperative arrhythmias

Advances in surgical treatment in the past one or two generations have transformed the outlook of many cardiovascular malformations from near-universal early mortality to one in which long-term survival is the norm and perioperative mortality is very low. We are now in the situation where there are more adults than children with congenital heart defects in the population. Most operations have evolved or changed completely over the years and part of the stimulus for this has been the desire to reduce late mortality and, notably, morbidity caused by late arrhythmia. It seems probable that the outlook for infants undergoing surgery now will be much better in the long run than it was for those 10 or 20 years ago, and the burden of late arrhythmia is likely to diminish significantly.

However, there are many patients under follow-up after surgery who are at risk of late arrhythmia, especially those who underwent a Mustard or Senning operation for transposition of the great arteries, those who had a Fontan operation, and those who had repair of a tetralogy of Fallot. The main arrhythmias of concern are incisional atrial tachycardia (atrial flutter), sinoatrial disease, and ventricular tachycardia.

Arrhythmias after the Senning and Mustard operations

Patients born with transposition of the great arteries in the 1970s and 1980s mostly underwent an atrial baffle repair – a Mustard or Senning operation. In the long run, most of them will develop arrhythmias, which contribute significantly to late morbidity and mortality and were one of the reasons for the change to the arterial switch operation 20 or so years ago. There is still a large population of young adult patients who underwent Mustard or Senning operations for transposition, and management of their arrhythmias presents a significant challenge. With time many patients lose sinus rhythm and develop a nodal or junctional bradycardia. This is not necessarily associated with symptoms and may not need intervention. If the patient is symptomatic, has marked bradycardia or pauses, or has significantly impaired systemic ventricular function, there may well be an indication for permanent pacemaker implantation.

Figure 32.1 shows a strip from an ambulatory ECG recording from a 23-year-old man who had had a Senning operation. It shows sinus bradycardia during waking hours, evidence of sinus node dysfunction (see Chapter 30). He had no symptoms, no tricuspid regurgitation, and fairly normal right ventricular function, so there was no indication for pacing.

Concise Guide to Pediatric Arrhythmias, First Edition. Christopher Wren.
© 2012 John Wiley & Sons, Ltd. Published 2012 by John Wiley & Sons, Ltd.

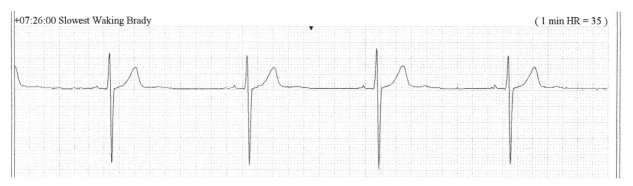

Figure 32.1

Figure 32.2 is another Holter recording from a young man who had previously had a Senning operation. It shows a prolonged sinus pause during sleep. He was well with few symptoms but had fairly profound bradycardia at other times on the recording, impaired right ventricular function, and moderate tricuspid regurgitation, and he did undergo pacemaker implantation. However, there is no good evidence that pacing reduces the risk of sudden death or atrial arrhythmias.

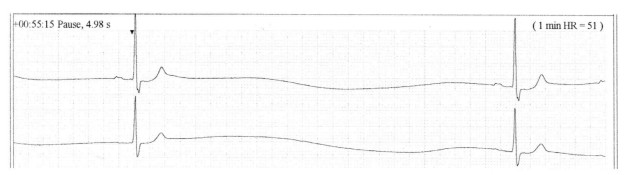

Figure 32.2

The most common and most significant tachycardia encountered is atrial flutter, also known as incisional atrial tachycardia. It is more common in patients with impaired systemic ventricular function. It may present with symptoms or may be an incidental finding on routine clinic review if the ventricular rate is not much affected.

Figure 32.3 is a rhythm strip from a 19-year-old man who had a Senning operation. It shows what is a normal QRS for him with a high ventricular rate with no discernable P waves. The diagnosis became clear when he was given intravenous adenosine. Atrioventricular (AV) conduction slows and the flutter waves are then obvious, before conduction settles down at 2:1.

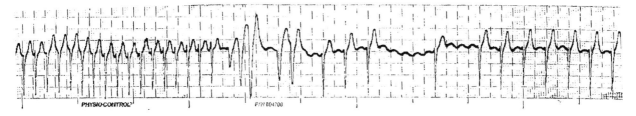

Figure 32.3

Figure 32.4 shows the heart rate trend from a 25-year-old man who attended clinic for routine follow-up. His ECG was thought to show sinus rhythm but his heart rate during waking hours was always 110/min, falling a little only when he was asleep (very unlike the normal heart rate variation seen in sinus rhythm). Closer inspection of the ECG confirmed atrial tachycardia with 2:1 AV conduction.

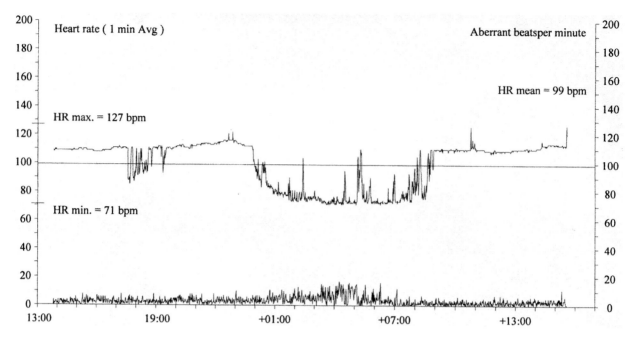

Figure 32.4

Figure 32.5 is from a 20-year-old woman who underwent a Senning operation. She developed sudden palpitation and breathlessness and her ECG shows a slightly irregular tachycardia of around 130/min which, at first glance in lead V1, might be mistaken for sinus rhythm. Closer inspection shows that she does not have normal P waves in other leads and the appearance in inferior leads suggests atrial flutter or tachycardia. The diagnosis was very clear on a second ECG recorded a few minutes later, showing atrial tachycardia at around 300/min with variable AV conduction (Figure 32.6).

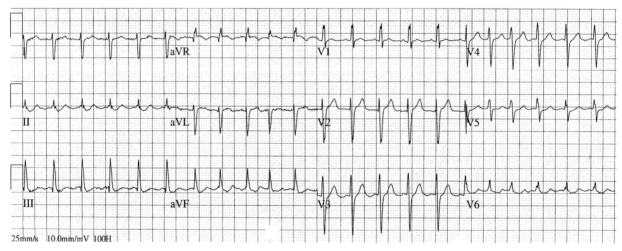

Figure 32.5

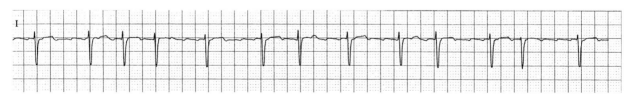

Figure 32.6

Acute management of atrial flutter in this situation involves DC cardioversion. Options for longer-term management include drug treatment for rate control and catheter ablation which has a reasonable success rate in expert hands.

The other significant problem after atrial repair of transposition is late sudden death. The risk is around 5 per 1000 patient-years, or a risk of 1 in 200 per year. Individual risk prediction is difficult but patients with poor cardiac function are at significantly higher risk. Death is very probably due to ventricular fibrillation or ventricular tachycardia, but identification of individuals at a high enough risk to recommend defibrillator implantation remains a challenge.

Arrhythmias after repair of a tetralogy of Fallot

Significant arrhythmias are uncommon in the early years after repair of a tetralogy of Fallot but they become increasingly prevalent late on. When they do occur they are often related to significant haemodynamic abnormalities, such as pulmonary regurgitation, impaired right ventricular function, and tricuspid regurgitation. The most common arrhythmias are atrial tachycardias (flutter or fibrillation) and ventricular tachycardia. If the QRS shows a pattern similar to right bundle branch block (RBBB) the diagnosis is almost certainly an atrial arrhythmia. If it shows left bundle branch block (LBBB) it is very probably ventricular tachycardia.

Incisional atrial re-entry tachycardia (atrial flutter) is probably the most common arrhythmia late after repair of tetralogy of Fallot. In Figure 32.7, from a young adult with repaired tetralogy of Fallot, there is an atrial tachycardia with 1:1 AV conduction and the RBBB pattern is a normal QRS for this patient.

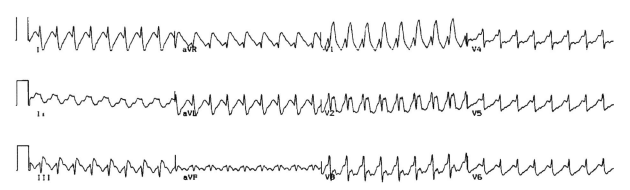

Figure 32.7

The diagnosis becomes clear only when conduction is reduced (Figure 32.8), when the P waves are visible (red arrows).

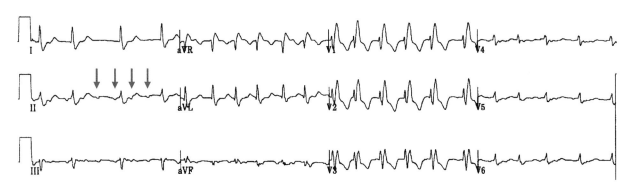

Figure 32.8

Figure 32.9 shows another example of atrial tachycardia late after repair of a tetralogy of Fallot. The clue to the diagnosis is the inappropriate heart rate of 160/min. Adenosine administration produces Wenckebach AV block without changing the atrial rate (arrows).

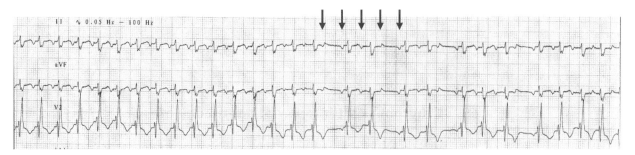

Figure 32.9

Atrial tachycardia usually occurs in patients with poor right ventricular function, often with pulmonary and/or tricuspid regurgitation. Acute treatment is best aimed at restoration of sinus rhythm with DC cardioversion. Options for longer-term management include drug treatment (with amiodarone, sotalol, etc.), catheter ablation, or surgery. If pulmonary valve replacement is planned, with or without tricuspid valve repair, it is advisable to perform a right atrial maze at the same time to reduce the risk of recurrence of atrial tachycardia.

Sustained ventricular tachycardia late after repair of a tetralogy of Fallot is a rare but serious problem. It may present with syncope, presyncope, palpitation, or breathlessness. The QRS pattern is usually similar to LBBB, as in Figure 32.10.

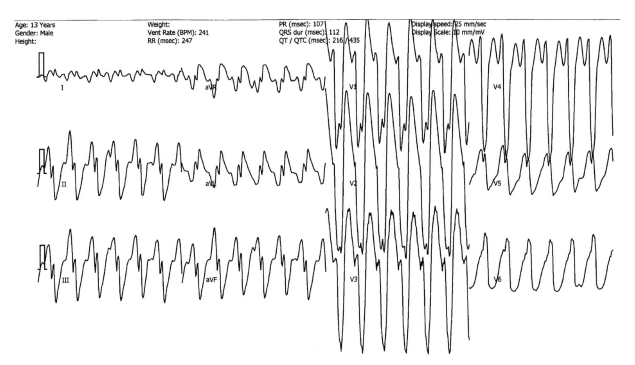

Figure 32.10

Figure 32.11 shows another example of ventricular tachycardia late after repair of a tetralogy of Fallot. The QRS is very broad with an inferior axis and a pattern resembling LBBB, suggesting that the origin of the arrhythmia is in the right ventricular outflow. The ECG pattern in a subsequent clinical episode of ventricular tachycardia

(VT) or after induction at an invasive electrophysiology study may show a different pattern because the re-entry circuits in these patients can be variable and complex.

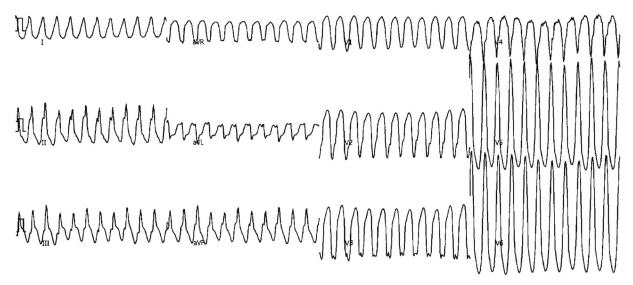

Figure 32.11

The treatment of VT depends mainly on the presence or absence of associated hemodynamic abnormalities. The acute management usually requires urgent DC cardioversion before planning a longer-term strategy. If pulmonary regurgitation makes pulmonary valve replacement necessary, the best option is preoperative or intraoperative electrophysiological mapping and intraoperative cryoablation of the arrhythmia circuit. Other options for treatment include antiarrhythmic drugs, catheter ablation, and defibrillator implantation.

Sudden death is rare late after repair of tetralogy of Fallot. The overall risk is around 1.5 per 1000 patient-years, or 1 in 700 per year. Although many "risk factors" have been proposed, none is useful prospectively, with the possible exception of transient AV block lasting for more than 3 days postoperatively. However, patients with syncope or sustained VT are probably at increased risk, and investigation and treatment will probably reduce the risk overall.

Arrhythmias after the Fontan operation

The Fontan operation and its variants offer definitive palliation for a variety of cardiovascular malformations with either a single or a common AV valve or a single or hypoplastic ventricle. The surgery has evolved rapidly over the past 20 years or so, and now usually comprises a staged approach culminating in a total cavopulmonary connection with an extracardiac conduit to connect the inferior vena cava to the pulmonary arteries. Recent modifications of the surgery are almost certainly associated with a significantly reduced risk of late arrhythmia but there are many adult patients surviving with a so-called "classic" Fontan circulation – with a direct atriopulmonary connection. Late arrhythmia is common in this situation and usually involves loss of sinus rhythm with bradycardia or incisional atrial macro re-entry tachycardia, otherwise commonly known as atrial flutter. The substrate for tachycardia is provided by right atrial dilation and hypertrophy plus scarring from previous surgery.

The ECG in Figure 32.12 comes from a 7-year-old boy with a total cavopulmonary connection. It shows a tachycardia of 260/min with a 1:1 AV relationship. P waves are clearly seen, being biphasic in lead I, negative in II and III, and positive in V1. On this ECG alone it is not easy to distinguish this from AV re-entry.

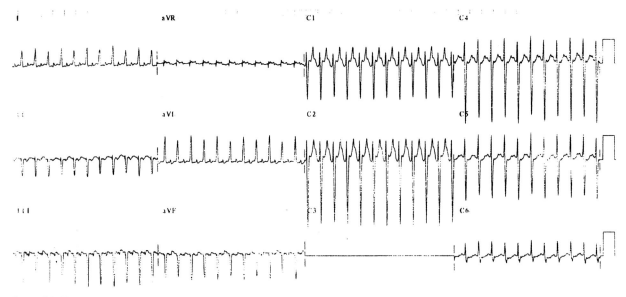

Figure 32.12

A second recording shown in Figure 32.13, taken a few minutes later, shows the same features but with 2:1 AV conduction. Accessory pathways cannot show 2:1 conduction in tachycardia so the diagnosis of atrial tachycardia is confirmed.

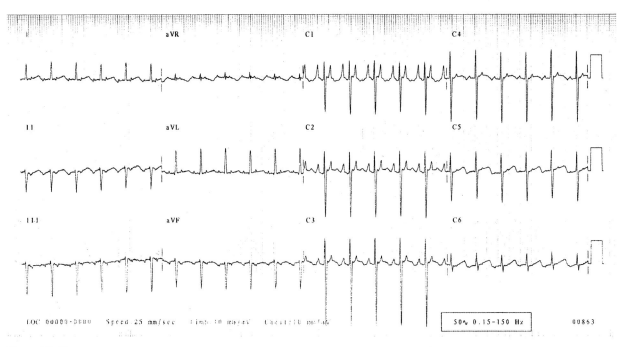

Figure 32.13

The ECG in Figure 32.14 is from a 15-year-old boy with tricuspid atresia and an atriopulmonary Fontan circulation. He was subject to very frequent episodes of tachycardia. The ECG shows a 1:1 AV relationship with a long PR interval and giant P waves characteristic of tricuspid atresia (arrows). Atrial tachycardia with 1:1 AV conduction should be strongly suspected from the history and the ECG. If the diagnosis was not certain it would be made clear by administration of adenosine, which will reduce AV conduction transiently (see Chapter 6).

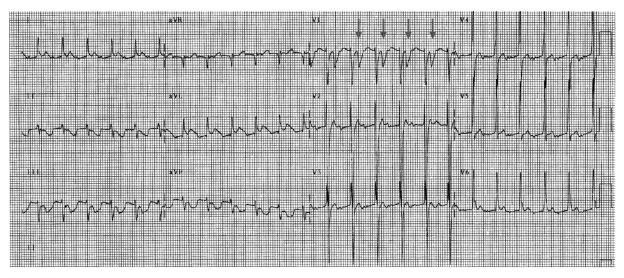

Figure 32.14

However, in this case adenosine was not necessary because the diagnosis was confirmed by the spontaneous development of 2:1 AV conduction as shown in Figure 32.15.

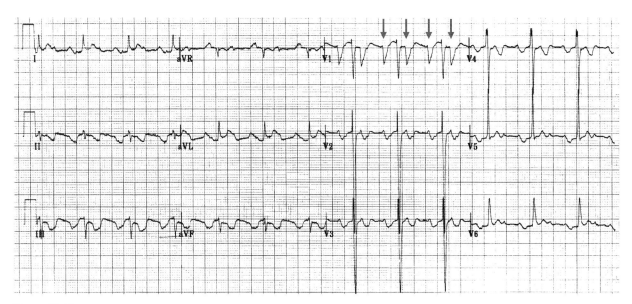

Figure 32.15

If the episode of atrial tachycardia is new it should be treated with DC cardioversion. If there are recurrences of tachycardia and it turns out to be a longer-term problem there are several management options. Antiarrhythmic drugs can be used in an attempt to prevent recurrence of tachycardia whereas long-term rate control is a less satisfactory option. Amiodarone is probably most often used but its use is associated with significant side effects in this population (see Chapter 37). Catheter ablation is sometimes used but has a fairly low success rate because of the nature and complexity of the substrate (see Chapter 39). The right atrium in patients with an atriopulmonary connection is often very dilated and hypertrophied with adherent mural thrombus. There may be multiple re-entry circuits. Catheter ablation in patients with newer versions of the Fontan circulation such as a lateral right atrial tunnel or an extracardiac conduit can be difficult or impossible if there is no venous access to the heart. Surgical conversion to a total cavopulmonary connection with a radical right atriectomy and biatrial maze operation is a very effective operation for some patients with a classic Fontan operation. It provides an additional significant hemodynamic improvement but is usually indicated only if there is troublesome recurrent tachycardia.

Pacing may be indicated for coexisting bradycardia but presents technical difficulties (see Chapter 38). In most patients with a Fontan circulation epicardial pacing is employed to avoid pacing leads within the systemic atrium and/or ventricle.

Other diagnoses

Arrhythmias are encountered in other malformations or diagnoses but less commonly than in the three discussed above. They are also an intrinsic feature of some malformation, as discussed in Chapter 33. Atrial arrhythmias are seen most commonly, usually with atrial enlargement, atrial hypertension, and previous atrial surgery providing the substrate. Figure 32.16 shows the ECG from a 7-year-old girl with severe mitral regurgitation in Beale's syndrome. She had preoperative atrial arrhythmias and developed incessant atrial tachycardia some months after a mitral valve repair and left atrial maze operation. She required two left atrial catheter ablation procedures before her arrhythmia was abolished. The ECG shows an atrial rate of 280/min with 2:1 AV conduction. The conducted P waves are easy to see (black arrows) and there is a prolonged PR interval. The non-conducted P waves are merged with the start of the QRS complexes and are less obvious at first sight (red arrows).

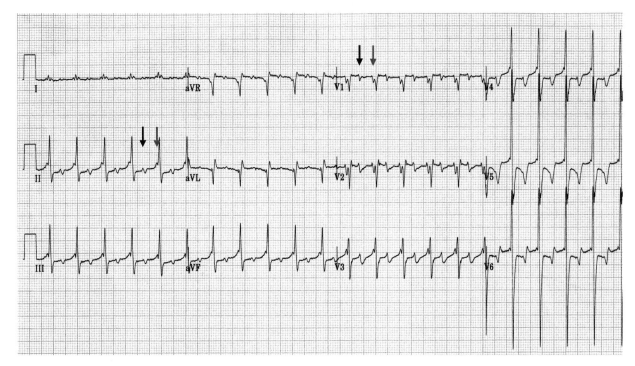

Figure 32.16

Figure 32.17 shows the ECG from a 15-year-old boy who had a biventricular repair of pulmonary atresia with intact ventricular septum in infancy and had been in atrial tachycardia for many years. He has also atrial tachycardia with 2:1 AV conduction but this is not immediately obvious. The conducted P waves are easily seen (black arrows) but the non-conducted P waves are partially hidden by the QRS (red arrows) and just appear as a pseudo second R wave. The diagnosis is suspected from the inappropriate ventricular rate and prolonged PR interval in this ECG, and the patient will also show a constant heart rate on ambulatory recording. If there is any doubt, ambulatory recording may also show higher-grade block or this can be produced with adenosine (see Chapter 6).

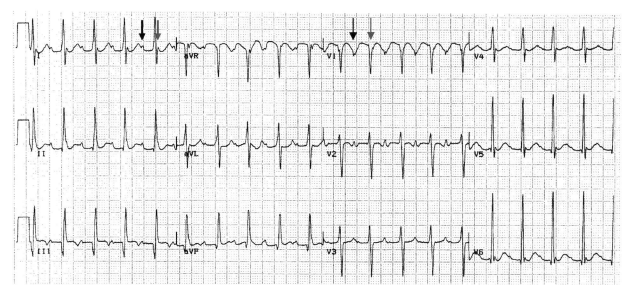

Figure 32.17

Figure 32.18 shows the ECG ventricular tachycardia in a 14-year-old boy who had previously undergone a Rastelli operation for complex transposition. He presented with syncope and was in this arrhythmia when he reached hospital. He was cardioverted into sinus rhythm and investigated with an electrophysiology study at which his arrhythmia was not inducible. He had no significant residual hemodynamic problem and was given an implanted defibrillator. He has had no appropriate shocks in 9 years of follow-up but several inappropriate shocks for atrial tachycardia.

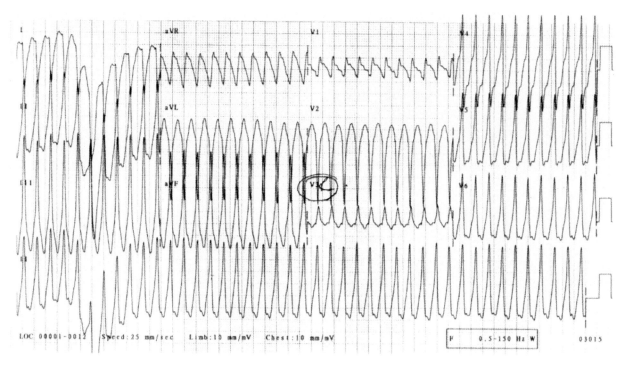

Figure 32.18

Key references

Deal BJ, Mavroudis C, Backer CL. Arrhythmia management in the Fontan patient. *Pediatr Cardiol* 2007;**28**:448–56.

Gatzoulis MA, Balaji S, Webber SA, et al. Risk factors for arrhythmia and sudden cardiac death late after repair of tetralogy of Fallot: a multicentre study. *Lancet* 2000;**356**:975–81.

Harrison DA, Siu SC, Hussain F, et al. Sustained atrial arrhythmias in adults late after repair of tetralogy of Fallot. *Am J Cardiol* 2001;**87**:584–8.

Kanter RJ, Garson A Jr. Atrial arrhythmias during chronic follow-up of surgery for complex congenital heart disease. *Pacing Clin Electrophysiol* 1997;**20**:502–11.

Mavroudis C, Deal BJ, Backer CL, et al. 111 Fontan conversions with arrhythmia surgery: surgical lessons and outcomes. *Ann Thorac Surg* 2007;**84**:1457–65.

Morwood JG, Triedman JK, Berul CI, et al. Radiofrequency catheter ablation of ventricular tachycardia in children and young adults with congenital heart disease. *Heart Rhythm* 2004;**1**:301–8.

Schwerzmann M, Salehian O, Harris L, et al. Ventricular arrhythmias and sudden death in adults after a Mustard operation for transposition of the great arteries. *Eur Heart J* 2009;**30**:1873–9.

Snyder CS. Postoperative ventricular tachycardia in patients with congenital heart disease: diagnosis and management. *Nature Rev Cardiol* 2008;**5**,469–76.

Stephenson EA, Lu M, Berul CI, et al. Arrhythmias in a contemporary Fontan cohort: prevalence and clinical associations in a multicenter cross-sectional study. *J Am Coll Cardiol* 2010;**56**:890–6.

Triedman JK. Arrhythmias in adults with congenital heart disease. *Heart* 2002;**87**:383–9.

Walsh EP, Cecchin F. Arrhythmias in adult patients with congenital heart disease. *Circulation* 2007;**115**;534–45.

33 Arrhythmias in congenital heart defects

Although the substrate for some arrhythmias is congenital, children with isolated arrhythmias are not regarded as having congenital heart disease. Most arrhythmias occur in structurally normal hearts, but there are several associations between cardiovascular malformations and arrhythmias where knowledge of the anatomical diagnosis may help interpretation of the arrhythmia. Early and late postoperative arrhythmias are discussed elsewhere (see Chapters 31 and 32 respectively).

Congenitally corrected transposition of the great arteries

The development of complete atrioventricular (AV) block is part of the natural history of patients with congenitally corrected transposition of the great arteries, occurring in around 5% at birth and in up to 25% overall in the long term. The risk of development of AV block at the time of surgical repair is high. Other arrhythmias encountered during follow-up include atrial flutter, atrial tachycardia or atrial fibrillation (all more likely with additional abnormalities of impaired ventricular function or left AV valve dysfunction), and supraventricular arrhythmias associated with an accessory pathway.

The ECGs below document the development of AV block in a girl with congenitally corrected transposition. As a neonate (Figure 33.1) she was in sinus rhythm and by the age of 4 years (Figure 33.2) had developed complete AV block.

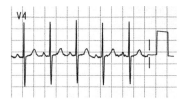

Figure 33.1

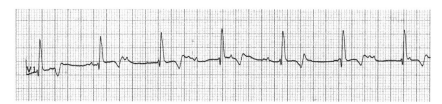

Figure 33.2

Concise Guide to Pediatric Arrhythmias, First Edition. Christopher Wren.
© 2012 John Wiley & Sons, Ltd. Published 2012 by John Wiley & Sons, Ltd.

Ebstein's anomaly of the tricuspid valve

Ebstein's anomaly of the tricuspid valve is probably the cardiovascular malformation most often associated with arrhythmias. These include AV re-entry tachycardia with an accessory pathway (usually right sided but not always with pre-excitation in sinus rhythm), AV nodal re-entry tachycardia, atriofascicular re-entry tachycardia, atrial flutter, atrial fibrillation, and, rarely, ventricular tachycardia. Accessory pathway arrhythmias are usually treated by radiofrequency ablation in older children and adults. Surgical repair of the tricuspid valve and/or the atrial septal defect may be combined with a right atrial maze procedure in the presence of atrial arrhythmias.

Figure 33.3 shows a 12-lead ECG from a boy with Ebstein's anomaly. The rhythm is sinus, with prominent respiratory sinus arrhythmia which produces variation in QRS morphology. At a slightly higher sinus rate there is a complex right bundle branch block (RBBB) pattern characteristic of Ebstein's malformation (black arrow). At a slightly lower rate there is ventricular pre-excitation with a pattern resembling left bundle branch block (LBBB) and characteristic of a right-sided accessory pathway (red arrow) – see Chapter 5. For one beat the right-sided bundle branch block and the right-sided pre-excitation cancel each other out and the QRS is normal (open arrow).

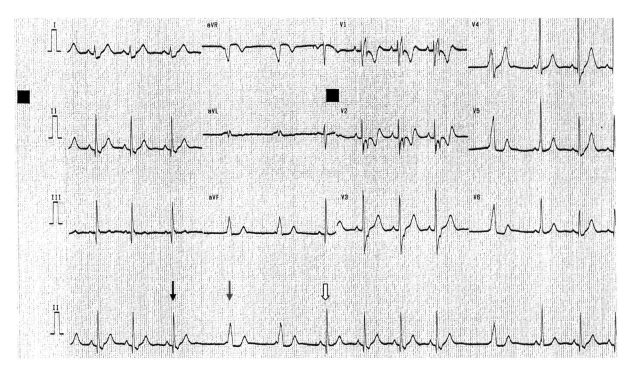

Figure 33.3

The ECG in Figure 33.4 shows AV re-entry tachycardia (AVRT) in a neonate with Ebstein's anomaly. The rate is around 230/min and the QRS shows right bundle branch block, which probably causes the tachycardia to run a little slower than usual for infant AVRT because the most likely substrate for the arrhythmia is a right-sided accessory pathway. The ECG in sinus rhythm showed the same QRS appearance, without ventricular pre-excitation.

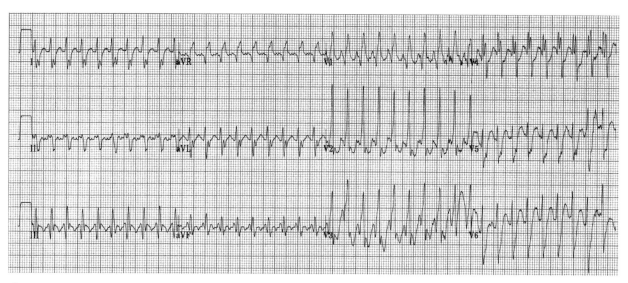

Figure 33.4

Atrial isomerism

In right atrial isomerism the heart has two sinus nodes and sometimes, depending on other structural abnormalities, two AV nodes. A variety of arrhythmias is reported, with "supraventricular tachycardia" being the most common. A rare arrhythmia is unique to this situation with AV re-entry caused by conduction down one AV node and back up the other. This can be elucidated only at invasive electrophysiological study.

In left atrial isomerism there is no true sinus node but the rhythm is usually atrial in origin. Atrial or junctional bradycardia is common but often does not require treatment. AV block may occur and has a poor prognosis if detected in fetal life.

Atrial septal defect

Arrhythmias are uncommon in children with isolated atrial septal defect but are common in adults. Atrial fibrillation and atrial flutter are the most commonly seen. Sinus node disease may be a feature of sinus venosus defects, with or without surgery. Arrhythmias occur in Holt Oram syndrome and other rare situations.

Key references

Anderson RH. The conduction tissues in congenitally corrected transposition. *Ann Thorac Surg* 2004;**77**:1881–2.

Bink-Boelkens MT, Bergstra A, Landsman ML. Functional abnormalities of the conduction system in children with an atrial septal defect. *Int J Cardiol* 1988;**20**:263–72.

Cheung YF, Cheng VY, Yung TC, et al. Cardiac rhythm and symptomatic arrhythmia in right atrial isomerism. *Am Heart J* 2002;**144**:159–64.

Connelly MS, Liu PP, Williams WG, et al. Congenitally corrected transposition of the great arteries in the adult: functional status and complications. *J Am Coll Cardiol* 1996;**27**:1238–43.

Delhaas T, du Marchie Sarvaas GJ, Rijlaarsdam ME, et al. A multicenter, long-term study on arrhythmias in children with Ebstein anomaly. *Pediatr Cardiol* 2010;**31**:229–33.

Khairy P, Dore A, Talajic M, et al. Arrhythmias in adult congenital heart disease. *Expert Rev Cardiovasc Ther* 2006;**4**:83–95.

Khositseth A, Danielson GK, Dearani JA, et al. Supraventricular tachyarrhythmias in Ebstein anomaly: management and outcome. *J Thorac Cardiovasc Surg* 2004;**128**:826–33.

34 Arrhythmias in cardiomyopathies

Hypertrophic cardiomyopathy

Hypertrophic cardiomyopathy is a dominantly inherited cardiac muscle disorder that produces myocyte and myofibrillar disorganization and fibrosis, with or without myocardial hypertrophy. These features are a potential substrate for arrhythmias. It is a rare diagnosis in childhood but is increasingly common in adult life. Clinical arrhythmias are also rare in children but there is a small risk of sudden death related to ventricular tachycardia. "Risk stratification" is poorly developed and prospective identification of children at significant risk is difficult.

Dilated cardiomyopathy

Dilated cardiomyopathy is associated with a variety of ventricular and supraventricular arrhythmias but arrhythmias appear not to influence the outcome. The overall risk of sudden death is low and adult indications for an implantable cardioverter/defibrillator (ICD) cannot be extrapolated to children.

Restrictive cardiomyopathy

This is a rare form of cardiomyopathy in children with a poor prognosis. The outcome is usually death or transplantation with a significant risk of sudden death from ventricular tachycardia or ventricular fibrillation. Atrioventricular (AV) block is also reported. Syncope is a poor prognostic sign and may be an indication for urgent listing for transplantation.

The ECGs in Figures 34.1 and 34.2 show the development of complete AV block in a 10-year-old boy with severe cardiomyopathy with some features of restrictive and some of hypertrophic cardiomyopathy. Figure 34.1 shows sinus rhythm with marked atrial hypertrophy (note that it is recorded at half gain). The PR interval is prolonged and there is left bundle branch block. He had a major syncopal episode and was found to have developed complete AV block (Figure 34.2 – recorded at standard gain). In some leads, notably II and V1, the P waves are larger than the QRS complexes.

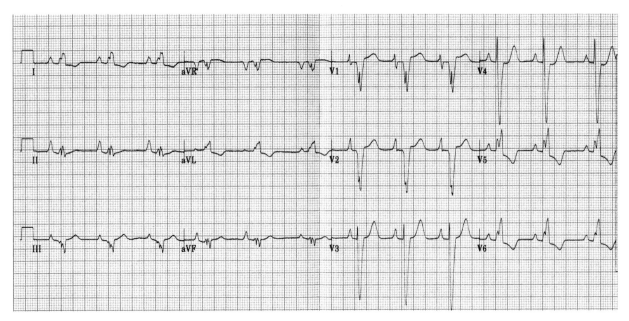

Figure 34.1

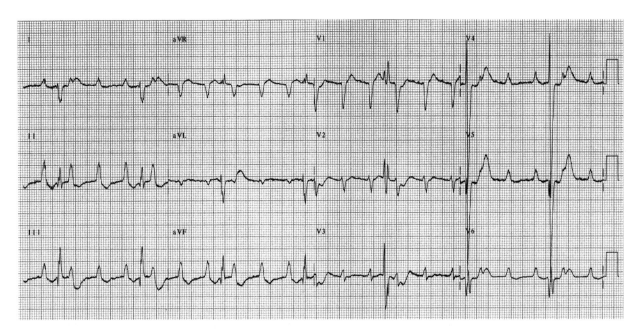

Figure 34.2

Kearns–Sayre syndrome

Kearns–Sayre syndrome is a rare mitochondrial myopathy characterized by ptosis, ophthalmoplegia, bilateral pigmentary retinopathy, and cardiac conduction abnormalities. The ECG will often show a bundle branch block and monitoring is required for any signs of progression to complete AV block. The ECG in Figure 34.3 is from a 16-year-old girl with Kearns–Sayre syndrome. It shows sinus rhythm with a normal PR interval, right bundle branch block, and left axis deviation. The ECG in Figure 34.4, recorded after the girl complained of increased lethargy, shows that she had developed complete AV block and required a permanent pacemaker.

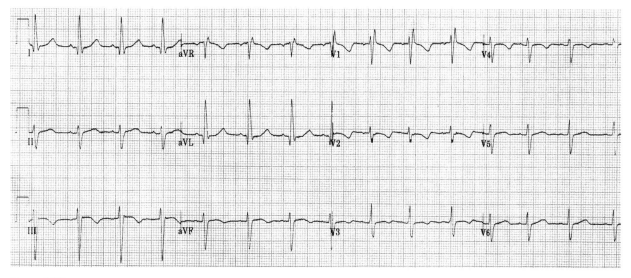

Figure 34.3

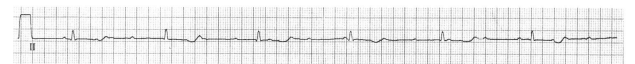

Figure 34.4

Duchenne muscular dystrophy

This is a severe recessive X-linked form of muscular dystrophy characterized by progressive muscle weakness, eventually leading to loss of ambulation and death. Cardiac involvement is present in almost all cases by later teenage. Atrial premature beats are common and the ECG may show a short PR interval. Clinically significant arrhythmias are rare.

Friedreich's ataxia

Friedreich's ataxia is an autosomal recessive congenital ataxia in which left ventricular hypertrophy is very common. Arrhythmias are unusual but atrial fibrillation and sinus tachycardia are reported.

Emery–Dreifuss muscular dystrophy

Emery–Dreifuss muscular dystrophy is a rare X-linked muscular dystrophy characterized by contractures, muscle weakness, and atrial arrhythmias. Sinoatrial disease with atrial tachycardias and junctional bradycardias is increasingly common during follow-up and pacemaker implantation is often indicated.

Becker muscular dystrophy

Becker muscular dystrophy is an X-linked recessively inherited disorder characterized by slowly progressive muscle weakness of the legs and pelvis. Conduction abnormalities are reported in adult patients.

Myotonic dystrophy

Arrhythmias are frequent in adults with myotonic dystrophy and may be associated with sudden death. Some patients require pacemaker or defibrillator implantation. Cardiac involvement in children is rare.

Barth's syndrome

Barth's syndrome is a rare X-linked cause of dilated cardiomyopathy in boys. It is also characterized by neutropenia, myopathy, and growth delay. It is sometimes associated with ventricular arrhythmias or sudden death. Diagnosis is confirmed by a biochemical cardiolipin assay.

Key references

Beynon RP, Ray SG. Cardiac involvement in muscular dystrophies. *Q J Med* 2008;**101**:337–44.

Dimas VV, Denfield SW, Friedman RA, et al. Frequency of cardiac death in children with idiopathic dilated cardiomyopathy. *Am J Cardiol* 2009;**104**:1574–7.

Pelargonio G, Dello Russo A, Sanna T, et al. Myotonic dystrophy and the heart. *Heart* 2002;**88**:665–70.

Rivenes SM, Kearney DL, Smith EO, et al. Sudden death and cardiovascular collapse in children with restrictive cardiomyopathy. *Circulation* 2000;**102**:876–82.

Sachdev B, Elliott PM, McKenna WJ. Cardiovascular complications of neuromuscular disorders. *Curr Treat Options Cardiovasc Med* 2002;**4**:171–9.

Spencer CT, Byrne BJ, Gewitz MH, et al. Ventricular arrhythmia in the X-linked cardiomyopathy Barth syndrome. *Pediatr Cardiol* 2005;**26**:632–7.

35 Syncope

Syncope is defined as a temporary loss of consciousness and postural tone secondary to a lack of adequate cerebral blood perfusion. It is a common problem, affecting up to 15–20% of children. Most of the many causes are benign but it is important to recognize the few that are potentially dangerous. Our understanding of syncope may be hindered by sometimes confusing terminology. Thus the most common group of causes, which includes the very common vasovagal syncope (simple fainting), is variously known as neurocardiogenic or reflex syncope. The main differential diagnosis of syncope is epilepsy and it is not always easy to tell them apart from the history alone (Table 35.1).

Table 35.1 Classification of syncope

Neurally mediated syncope (also known as reflex syncope)
Vasovagal syncope
Reflex asystolic syncope (also known as reflex anoxic seizures)
Orthostatic hypotension
Postural orthostatic tachycardia syndrome

Cardiac syncope
Structural malformation
Arrhythmia
Hypertrophic cardiomyopathy
Restrictive cardiomyopathy
Pulmonary hypertension

Non-cardiovascular syncope
Psychogenic syncope
Factitious syncope

Vasovagal syncope

By far the most common type of syncope in children, vasovagal syncope is caused by arterial and venous dilation associated with bradycardia. It is usually precipitated by a trigger, which may be physical (prolonged standing, hot environment, hair brushing, etc.) or emotional (having blood taken, watching video of medical procedures, etc.), but sometimes there is little or no warning. It may also occur shortly after exercise. Vasovagal syncope is usually preceded by a feeling of dizziness or lightheadedness, palpitation, partial loss of vision. and sweating. Recovery of consciousness usually occurs within a minute or two. If the child does not adopt, or is not put into, a recumbent or recovery position, unconsciousness may be prolonged and a secondary anoxic seizure may occur.

Concise Guide to Pediatric Arrhythmias, First Edition. Christopher Wren.
© 2012 John Wiley & Sons, Ltd. Published 2012 by John Wiley & Sons, Ltd.

Reflex asystolic syncope

Previously also known as reflex anoxic seizures or pallid breath-holding attacks, this is typically a problem of pre-school children with the onset of symptoms usually before the age of 2 years. Syncope is usually precipitated by a sudden shock, fright, bump, or disappointment, or other noxious stimulus. The toddler may emit a cry and then fall apparently lifeless, being very pale and unconscious. Reflex asystolic syncope is caused by prolonged asystole as shown on ambulatory monitoring in Figure 35.1. Although initially very frightening for parents, this type of syncope seems to be benign and usually resolves spontaneously before school age. Occasionally it may persist into the teens.

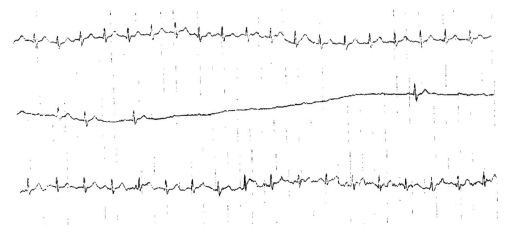

Figure 35.1

Orthostatic hypotension

Another relatively common type of syncope, this typically occurs a few moments after standing or while standing. It is more common in tall thin children and probably has a similar mechanism to vasovagal syncope. Orthostatic presyncope is even more common and is probably experienced by most children at some time.

Postural orthostatic tachycardia syndrome

Postural orthostatic tachycardia syndrome (POTS) is a recently recognized condition that may be diagnosed in older children. It is a heterogeneous group of disorders that result from disturbance of normal autonomic control. It is defined as the chronic presence of symptoms of orthostatic intolerance associated with a heart rate increase of 30/min (or rate that exceeds 120/min) within 10 min of standing or upright tilt, in the absence of any other cause. Presyncope is common but syncope is usually not a dominant feature. It has recently been suggested that POTS is due to a small stroke volume in patients with reduced left ventricular mass and can be improved by exercise training.

Psychogenic syncope

Psychogenic syncope is rare in younger children but less so in adolescent girls. The diagnosis is more likely if syncope is very frequent (daily or even more common) and is prolonged despite a supine posture. During an episode an unusual posture may be adopted and the eyes may be kept tightly closed. Despite the claimed frequency of symptoms, they usually fail to be reproduced during ambulatory ECG or blood pressure monitoring.

Structural cardiac abnormalities

Syncope is an uncommon presentation but may lead to diagnosis of conditions such as aortic valve stenosis or pulmonary hypertension. There are usually other symptoms and always abnormal signs on physical examination.

Cardiomyopathies

Syncope may be a feature of hypertrophic or restrictive cardiomyopathy, being an ominous sign in the latter. It may be caused by an arrhythmia such as complete atrioventricular (AV) block or ventricular tachycardia, or may result from hemodynamic factors such as the inability to increase the cardiac output because of left ventricular outflow tract obstruction, diastolic dysfunction, or myocardial ischemia.

Arrhythmias

A variety of arrhythmias may present with syncope, including ventricular tachycardia in long QT syndrome (see Chapter 25) or catecholaminergic polymorphic ventricular tachycardia (see Chapter 26), atrial fibrillation in Wolff–Parkinson–White syndrome (see Chapter 13), and complete AV block (see Chapter 29). The ECG in Figure 35.2 was recorded in a 12-year-old girl who presented after a single major syncopal episode and was found to have complete atrioventricular block. Although no cause for it could be proven, examination of her medical records revealed documentation of bradycardia on several occasions since the age of 12 months.

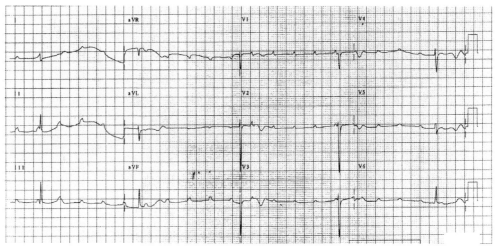

Figure 35.2

Investigation of syncope

Investigation will be guided by the history, which should ideally be first hand from a witness because the child may be too young or may not remember much about the event. Nearly all syncope is benign and requires limited investigation, but a history of syncope related to excitement, fright, exertion, or swimming may be a clue to a potentially dangerous underlying cause.

Unless there is a typical history of vasovagal syncope, most children reaching medical attention should have a 12-lead ECG, mainly to check that the QT interval is normal. The ECG may also show ventricular pre-excitation in Wolff–Parkinson–White syndrome (see Chapter 13) or complete AV block (see Chapter 29).

Tilt testing may be helpful in some children with recurrent syncope. The protocol varies but involves lying supine for at least 15 min and being tilted to 60–80° from the horizontal for up to 30–45 min. Tilt testing has a high false-positive and false-negative rate but can be helpful if typical symptoms are reproduced and accompanied by changes in heart rate and blood pressure (see Chapter 3).

An exercise ECG may be indicated if symptoms are related to exercise, although in practice it will usually be normal. A random 24-hour ambulatory ECG recording is also very likely to be normal because the likelihood of further symptoms occurring during recording is low. A loop recorder or event recorder can be worn for a longer time but is useful only if symptoms are fairly frequent. If a serious arrhythmia is suspected an implantable loop recorder may prove useful. It is implanted subcutaneously in the left axilla and can provide automatic or parent-activated recordings for up to 3 years.

The recording in Figure 35.3 is from an implanted loop recorder in a 10-year-old girl with infrequent but recurrent syncope. Her 12-lead ECG was normal but the rhythm during a syncopal episode clearly shows a prolonged episode of torsades de pointes (see also Chapter 25). Subsequent genetic analysis proved the presence long QT syndrome type 1.

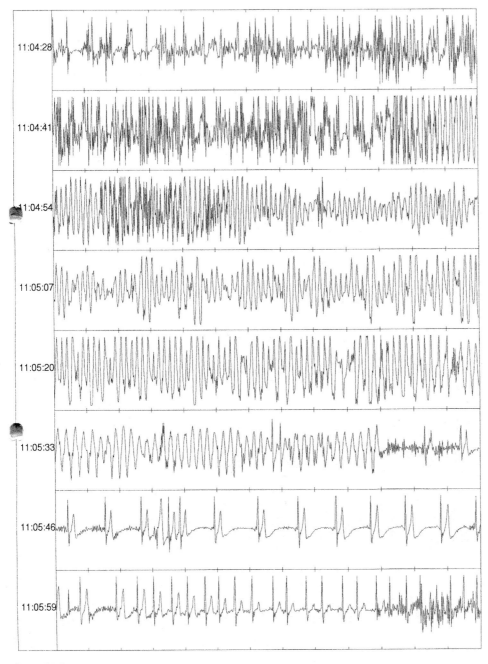

Figure 35.3

Management of syncope

Advice and management will obviously depend on the diagnosis. In most cases the mechanism of syncope is benign and the most important action is to give reassurance that the child does not have a serious heart problem or epilepsy and will not drop dead. In the most common situation of vasovagal syncope, advice can be given on how to prevent attacks by eating a regular normal diet and drinking plenty of fluids or by avoiding specific triggering situations. If there are prodromal symptoms, attacks may be aborted by lying down or by squatting or walking or tensing the abdominal muscles and crossing the legs. β-blocking or mineralocorticoid drugs are sometimes used but in trials may offer no benefit over a placebo. The efficacy of more aggressive drug treatment is often limited by severe side effects.

Reflex asystolic syncope in toddlers is difficult to prevent but parents should be instructed to put the child into the recovery position and to avoid picking him or her up. Various drug treatments have been tried but none is of proven benefit. In a few cases, when symptoms are frequent and severe, a permanent pacemaker may be considered.

Management of postural orthostatic tachycardia syndrome may involve avoidance of drugs that may precipitate or worsen attacks, physical exercise and reconditioning, increasing fluid and salt intake, and use of pharmacological agents.

Conclusion

Syncope is a common symptom in children and most causes are benign. A thorough history will help to identify the rare cases with a potentially serious underlying cause. Most children should have a 12-lead ECG and further investigation (if any) will depend on the history and the likely diagnosis.

Key references

Brady PA, Low PA, Shen WK. Inappropriate sinus tachycardia, postural orthostatic tachycardia syndrome, and overlapping syndromes. *PACE* 2005;**28**:1112–21.

Elliott P, McKenna W. The science of uncertainty and the art of probability. Syncope and its consequences in hypertrophic cardiomyopathy. *Circulation* 2009;**119**:1697–9.

Fu Q, VanGundy TB, Galbreath M, et al. Cardiac origins of the postural orthostatic tachycardia syndrome. *J Am Coll Cardiol* 2010;**55**:2858–68.

Grubb BP. Neurocardiogenic syncope and related disorders of orthostatic intolerance. *Circulation* 2005;**111**;2997–3006.

Grubb BP. Postural tachycardia syndrome. *Circulation* 2008;**117**;2814–17.

Massin MM, Bourguignont A, Coremans C, et al. Syncope in pediatric patients presenting to an emergency department. *J Pediatr* 2004;**145**;223–8.

McLeod KA. Syncope in childhood. *Arch Dis Child* 2003;**88**:350–3.

Mosqueda-Garcia R, Furlan R, Tank J, et al. The elusive pathophysiology of neurally mediated syncope. *Circulation* 2000;**102**;2898–906.

Steinberg LA, Knilans TK. Syncope in children: diagnostic tests have a high cost and low yield. *J Pediatr* 2005;**146**:355–8.

Wieling W, Ganzeboom KS, Saul JP. Reflex syncope in children and adolescents. *Heart* 2004;**90**:1094–100.

36 Sudden death

The sudden death of an apparently normal child is a rare event with a profound impact on parents, family, friends, and schoolmates. It often generates publicity and instills fear in the parents of other healthy children. If the autopsy reveals a previously unsuspected cardiac abnormality, this raises the question of whether it could have been detected and death might have been prevented. If no cause is found, and a cardiac arrhythmia is presumed to be responsible, there is no satisfactory resolution for the parents.

Specific data on the incidence of unexpected sudden death in children are not easy to find and probably underestimate the true figure. From various published reports it is reasonable to conclude that the overall risk of sudden cardiac death in apparently normal children is around 4–5 per 10^6 age-specific person-years or 1:200 000–1:250 000 per year. This represents about 4% of all deaths in this age group and equates to four or five deaths during school years for every 100 000 children.

Data on the causes of sudden death in children are lacking. Such data as are available come mainly from studies of populations up to 35 years of age. In published studies of deaths of young athletes in the United States of America and Italy, hypertrophic cardiomyopathy, premature coronary artery disease, arrhythmogenic right ventricular cardiomyopathy, congenital coronary anomalies, and myocarditis predominate. Few deaths were ascribed to ion channelopathies and very few had "normal" hearts. The number of sudden deaths with no explanation seems low in these reports, given the fact that most primary arrhythmias leave no trace after death. In children we would expect no deaths from premature coronary artery disease and very few from arrhythmogenic right ventricular cardiomyopathy. The main structural causes are likely to be hypertrophic cardiomyopathy and anomalous coronary arteries and a higher proportion is expected to be due to primary cardiac arrhythmias (leaving an apparently normal heart after death) (Table 36.1).

Hypertrophic cardiomyopathy is characterized by macroscopic left ventricular hypertophy and histological myocyte disarray. It is caused by a mutation in one of the genes that encode for sarcomere proteins and usually exhibits autosomal dominant inheritance. It is said to be a common disease in adults but is much less common in children. There are a few reports that enable us to estimate the risk of sudden death from previously undetected hypertrophic cardiomyopathy in childhood and during the teens at around 1 per 10^6 age-specific person-years. The individual risk is higher at younger ages and peaks below 14 years – the age at which screening is sometimes recommended. Most deaths occur at rest rather than during strenuous exertion.

Arrhythmogenic right ventricular cardiomyopathy is a rare disease in childhood and most sudden deaths reported are in young men. One report puts the sudden death rate at less than 1 per 10^6 age-specific person-years for those aged <20 years.

Anomalous origin of a coronary artery from the contralateral aortic sinus is probably not rare in the population. Coronary angiographic studies suggest a prevalence of around 0.5–1:1000 but such reports may exhibit ascertainment bias. The cumulative

Concise Guide to Pediatric Arrhythmias, First Edition. Christopher Wren.
© 2012 John Wiley & Sons, Ltd. Published 2012 by John Wiley & Sons, Ltd.

Table 36.1 Main potential causes of sudden cardiac death in children

Cause	Prevalence	Sudden death/10^6
Cardiomyopathy		
Hypertrophic cardiomyopathy	?1:10000	1
Arrhythmogenic right ventricular cardiomyopathy	Rare	?0.8
Cardiovascular malformation		
• Anomalous origin of a coronary artery	?1:2000	0.5
Primary arrhythmia		
Congenital long QT syndrome	?1:5000	?
Catecholaminergic polymorphic ventricular tachycardia	Rare	Rare
Wolff–Parkinson–White syndrome	1:700	Rare
Brugada syndrome	Rare	Rare
Other		
Myocarditis	–	0.5
Commotio cordis	–	Rare
Total	3:1000	4–5

lifetime risk is unknown. Sudden death from this cause has been estimated at 0.5 per 10^6 person-years meaning that the individual risk is fairly low.

As mentioned above, the number of apparently normal hearts in autopsy series is surprisingly low. Until recently, the coroner's pathologist's primary responsibility was to ensure that death was natural and it was not well recognized that unexplained sudden death in children is mainly due to primary cardiac arrhythmia. The most common cause of sudden death in children is probably *congenital long QT syndrome* (see Chapter 25). Gene mutations causing long QT syndrome are thought to be present in around 1 in 5000 in the population. The frequency with which long QT syndrome presents with sudden death is very difficult to assess because of the difficulty of retrospective diagnosis although recent reports of molecular autopsy have found significant numbers. *Catecholaminergic polymorphic ventricular tachycardia* is probably rare and is predominantly a disease of young children (see Chapter 26). *Brugada syndrome* is rare in children (see Chapter 27). *Wolff–Parkinson–White syndrome* is one of the most common causes of arrhythmia in childhood but sudden deaths are very rare (see Chapter 13).

Myocarditis is a rare confirmed clinical disease in life but is a consistent finding in reports of sudden deaths in young people. Population studies suggest an incidence of sudden death of around 0.5 per 10^6 age-specific person-years up to the age of 20 years.

Commotio cordis describes sudden death from ventricular fibrillation triggered by blunt trauma to the chest. As such it mainly represents extreme misfortune because there is no primary cardiac abnormality. It is a sporadic event and not amenable to prediction from screening. Over a third of cases occur outside competitive sports activities.

Family screening in the event of sudden death

After a sudden unexpected death there is a responsibility to offer assessment to other family members – usually only to first-degree relatives. It is important to obtain a complete pedigree to identify individuals likely to benefit from screening. The best approach is to use a stepwise assessment and to extend screening through the family only if other key individuals are identified. It is not appropriate to start with distant relatives – it is common for parents to ask for their children to be screened when they have not been assessed themselves. The assessment of the family depends fundamentally on the cause of sudden death. The autopsy should be able to provide confirmation of familial diseases such as hypertrophic cardiomyopathy, dilated cardiomyopathy, arrhythmogenic right ventricular cardiomyopathy, and aortic rupture in Marfan's syndrome, and to identify non-familial abnormalities such as coronary artery malformations. The autopsy will be unhelpful in primary electrical diagnoses such as long QT syndrome, catecholaminergic polymorphic ventricular tachycardia, Brugada syndrome.

Guided by the known cause of death, family screening of children may involve ECG, echocardiogram, ambulatory ECG, ajmaline or flecainide challenge, genetic analysis, etc. The most difficult, and one of the most common, clinical situations encountered is sudden death from no known cause in a family member. What screening of children in the family should be recommended in this situation? A detailed history, clinical examination, ECG, and echocardiogram seem sensible recommendations for all children who are first-degree relatives. The echocardiogram is likely to be unhelpful if the autopsy was normal, because that will already have excluded cardiomyopathy, Marfan's syndrome, etc. as a cause of death. The ECG will be helpful to measure a normal QT interval but can be normal in some long QT gene carriers and is likely to be normal in carriers of genes for catecholaminergic polymorphic ventricular tachycardia or Brugada syndrome.

Sudden death related to swimming, and not thought to be related simply to drowning, seems often to be fairly specific for some sorts of cardiac channel defects. In particular, investigations have shown a high probability of the finding of long QT syndrome type 1 or catecholaminergic polymorphic ventricular tachycardia in this situation. The ECG is very likely to be able to predict the presence of long QT syndrome. In some circumstances, when the ECG is normal, it may be felt appropriate to offer exercise ECG testing or genetic screening for catecholaminergic polymorphic ventricular tachycardia.

Population screening

Published guidelines in Europe and the USA recommend screening of "young competitive athletes" from the age of 14 years. Although there would undeniably be a potential benefit from early diagnosis of some primary arrhythmias such as long QT syndrome if screening were introduced, the benefit of presymptomatic diagnosis of other diseases such as hypertrophic cardiomyopathy, Wolff–Parkinson–White syndrome, or coronary artery anomalies is unproven. Current recommendations for screening, if implemented, would probably detect fewer than half of children potentially at risk because they target the wrong diagnoses, the wrong age groups, and focus on "athletes", when all children take part in strenuous exercise. More specific information on the prevalence and spectrum of latent cardiac disease in children is needed before screening can be recommended.

Key references

Bardai A, Berdowski J, van der Werf C, et al. Incidence, causes, and outcomes of out-of-hospital cardiac arrest in children: a comprehensive, prospective, population-based study in the Netherlands. *J Am Coll Cardiol* 2011;**57**:1822–8.

Basso C, Maron BJ, Corrado C, et al. Clinical profile of congenital coronary arteries with origin from the wrong aortic sinus leading to sudden death in young competitive athletes. *J Am Coll Cardiol* 2000;**35**:1493–501.

Elliott PM, Poloniecki J, Dickie S, et al. Sudden death in hypertrophic cardiomyopathy: identification of high risk patients. *J Am Coll Cardiol* 2000;**36**:2212–18.

Maron BJ, Gohman TE, Kyle SB, et al. Clinical profile and spectrum of commotio cordis. *JAMA* 2002;**287**:1142–6.

Pelliccia A. The preparticipation cardiovascular screening of competitive athletes: is it time to change the customary clinical practice? *Eur Heart J* 2007;**28**:2703–5.

van der Werf C, van Langen IM, Wilde AAM. Sudden death in the young: what do we know about it and how to prevent? *Circ Arrhythm Electrophysiol* 2010;**3**:96–104.

Wren C. Sudden death in children and adolescents. *Heart* 2002;**88**:426–31.

Wren C. Screening children with a family history of sudden death. *Heart* 2006;**92**:1001–6.

Wren C. Screening for potentially fatal heart disease in children and teenagers. *Heart* 2009;**95**:2040–6.

37 Antiarrhythmic drug treatment

Despite recent developments in treatment of tachycardias, particularly the development of catheter ablation, antiarrhythmic drugs continue to play an important role in the acute and chronic treatment of arrhythmias in children. The actions of the drugs are similar in adults and children but there are important differences, both in the arrhythmia substrate and in the child's metabolism of the drug.

Introduction of new drugs into pediatric practice has been cautious and usually follows evidence of efficacy in adults. Very few antiarrhythmic drugs are specifically licensed for use in children. It is obviously important for any pediatrician or cardiologist prescribing a drug to be familiar with details of dosage, effects, and adverse effects. A brief summary of the important information on some commonly used antiarrhythmic drugs follows. For more details consult a pediatric formulary.

The method of assessment of efficacy of treatment depends on the arrhythmia being treated. Control of paroxysmal tachycardias in children can be judged from the absence of symptoms. The aim of treatment of incessant tachycardias in children may be suppression of the arrhythmia or rate control and is often best assessed by ambulatory ECG monitoring.

Adenosine

The electrophysiological effects of adenosine include slowing of atrioventricular (AV) node conduction and suppression of sinus node automaticity. It also shortens atrial refractoriness but has little effect on ventricular myocardium. Clinically its predominant effect is on the AV node and use is made of this in the diagnosis and treatment of tachycardia. The AV node is a right atrial structure and adenosine also has significant clinical effects on some atrial arrhythmias and may suppress the sinus node. When given in sinus rhythm it may cause sinus bradycardia or atrial bradycardia or AV block. A few rare types of ventricular tachycardia are also suppressed by adenosine.

Adenosine is metabolized by red blood cells and its half-life is very short. As a result of this it has to be given by rapid bolus injection in a sufficient dose to reach the coronary circulation (the blood supply to the AV node) from a peripheral intravenous injection. Doses can be repeated with no cumulative effect.

Indications

Intravenous adenosine is the first-line treatment for any sustained regular tachycardia in infancy or childhood, with either a normal or a wide QRS. Adenosine is not recommended for sustained *irregular* tachycardias, partly because the mechanism of the arrhythmia should already be apparent from analysis of the ECG and partly because there is the possibility of producing hemodynamic deterioration from acceleration of the ventricular rate (see below). Adenosine is not helpful in the treatment of intermittent tachycardias because its effect is so short lasting.

Dosing

When the first clinical investigations of adenosine were performed in children in the 1980s the appropriate dose was not known. As a result of this early studies used a stepwise incremental dose strategy, starting from 37.5 or 50 μg/kg with similar increments. Unfortunately these experimental protocols continued into recent guidelines for dosing, despite many reports of the lack of efficacy of smaller doses. Adenosine doses of 50 μg/kg are rarely effective and 100 μg/kg is also often ineffective, especially in infancy. Around a third of infants and two-thirds of children respond to a dose of 150 μg/kg.

Administration

The first dose of 150 μg/kg is given as a bolus via an intravenous cannula fitted with a three-way tap so the adenosine injection can be followed by a rapid flush of physiological (0.9%) saline or dextrose. The ECG should be recorded during administration (preferably three leads – I, aVF, and V1) as well as a 12-lead ECG before and after. It is not adequate simply to observe the ECG on a monitor because termination of tachycardia, even if only temporary, will provide important diagnostic information. If the first dose is ineffective, the second should be 50 or 100 μg/kg higher.

Clinical effects

The clinical use of adenosine takes advantage of its dominant effect of slowing AV conduction. Many common types of "supraventricular" tachycardia involve re-entry through the AV node which is a fundamental part of the arrhythmia circuit. Such arrhythmias are reliably terminated by adenosine, because they cannot continue in the presence of AV nodal block.

The effect of adenosine on atrial arrhythmias is less predictable. It will not terminate atrial flutter but does cause impairment of AV conduction to unmask the flutter. This can be a great help in diagnosis if 1:1 or 2:1 AV conduction makes precise diagnosis difficult. The effect on other atrial arrhythmias varies. Atrial ectopic tachycardia may be unmasked by showing 2:1 conduction but may also be transiently suppressed, making differential diagnosis from sinus tachycardia more difficult. Rarer re-entry tachycardias (such as permanent junctional reciprocating tachycardia or atriofascicular re-entry tachycardia) are usually terminated, if only transiently, but require specialist assessment. Adenosine rarely terminates ventricular tachycardia but careful analysis of the ECG during administration may identify production of retrograde block (see Chapter 6).

Adverse effects

Side effects of adenosine, such as flushing, dyspnea, or chest pain, are common but are fleeting and usually minor. It is worth warning older children of these before adenosine is given.

Although warnings or contraindications to use in asthma are commonly given, there is no evidence that adenosine causes clinical problems in children with asthma and good evidence that it does not do so in adults.

Transient bradycardia after termination of tachycardia with adenosine is common but significant proarrhythmia is rare, especially in children. One situation to be aware of is the possibility of increasing AV conduction when giving adenosine to a patient with atrial flutter and 2:1 AV conduction. The sympathetic response to transient systemic vasodilation and mild hypotension induced by adenosine can occasionally increase AV conduction to 1:1, which may cause hemodynamic compromise.

Adenosine is also widely used during invasive investigation of arrhythmias in the electrophysiology laboratory using, for example, its effect on the AV node to unmask accessory pathways (which are mainly unaffected by adenosine).

Amiodarone

Amiodarone is an antiarrhythmic drug with complex actions. It is effective in treatment of many types of tachycardia but has more significant adverse effects than most of the other antiarrhythmic drugs that we use. As a result of this its use is often restricted to persistent difficult tachycardias.

Indications

Amiodarone is used for treatment of a wide variety of arrhythmias. In infants it is effective in controlling AV re-entry tachycardia (AVRT) and side effects are few. It also controls infant permanent junctional reciprocating tachycardia and congenital junctional ectopic tachycardia, and other incessant tachycardias.

Beyond infancy amiodarone is mainly used for control of difficult atrial or ventricular arrhythmias, particularly in older children or young adults with repaired congenital cardiac malformations.

Intravenous amiodarone is used to gain acute control of incessant arrhythmias in the intensive care unit. It may be effective against postoperative junctional ectopic tachycardia, atrial ectopic tachycardia, and rare types of ventricular tachycardia.

Dosing

Dosing regimens for intravenous amiodarone vary. A loading dose of 5 mg/kg over 30 min or 5 mg/kg divided into four bolus doses in the first hour is usually given. As a result of concerns that amiodarone may cause plastic to leach from intravenous tubing at low infusion rates, maintenance administration is often given as a series of equally divided boluses, each infused every few hours over 10 min.

Because of concerns over potential side effects of intravenous treatment (see below), oral loading doses are preferred, unless an immediate effect is required or the patient cannot take oral medication. A loading dose of 15 mg/kg per day is usually effective in infants and younger children, reducing after 10 days to a maintenance dose of 5–10 mg/kg per day. In older children and young adults the loading dose can be 200 mg three times daily reducing after 1 week to 100 or 200 mg daily, depend on the effect.

Clinical effects

The method of judging the efficacy of treatment depends on the arrhythmia. With some tachycardias, such as AVRT or postoperative atrial tachycardia, the aim will be complete suppression of tachycardia. With others, such as junctional ectopic tachycardia, rate control is often a reasonable objective. Ambulatory ECG monitoring will often be employed to confirm the effectiveness of treatment.

Adverse effects

Acute adverse effects seen with intravenous treatment include hypotension, vomiting, bradycardia, and AV block. Most are dose-related and temporary. Problems with chronic oral administration include photosensitivity (which can be controlled by sunblock), skin discoloration, corneal microdeposits, disturbance of liver function tests, pneumonitis, and hyper- or hypothyroidism but such complications are rare in infancy. Most are reversible if treatment is withdrawn. Most texts recommend periodic monitoring of liver, thyroid, and lung function in patients on long-term treatment outside infancy.

Amiodarone interacts with a number of other drugs including warfarin, digoxin, and flecainide, and dose adjustment will usually be necessary.

β-Blockers

Several β-blocking drugs are used in treatment of pediatric arrhythmias, the most common being propranolol, atenolol, nadolol, sotalol, and esmolol. β-Blockers form the mainstay of treatment for some conditions such as congenital long QT syndrome and catecholaminergic polymorphic ventricular tachycardia. They are also commonly used for paroxysmal supraventricular arrhythmias, perhaps being more effective in suppression of AV nodal re-entry tachycardia than AV re-entry. β-Blockers are less effective in control of incessant tachycardias such as atrial ectopic tachycardia and junctional ectopic tachycardia.

To some extent the choice of β-blocker depends on personal preference because there is little evidence of differing activity against various arrhythmias. They share common side effects. Weariness or fatigue is common at the start of treatment but usually not a major problem. Some children experience cold extremities or sleep disturbance (the latter may be less frequent with atenolol or sotalol). Worsening or precipitation of asthma is a potential problem but the risk is probably overstated. Where there is no alternative (as, for example, in long QT syndrome) a β-blocker can often be introduced under close clinical supervision without major problems.

Propranolol
Propranolol is the β-blocker with which there is the greatest clinical experience. Its main drawback is its short half-life which makes more frequent administration necessary. It is mainly used orally in a dose of around 3 mg/kg per day in three or four doses. Tablets of 10, 40, and 80 mg are available. Oral solutions of various concentrations are available for smaller children. It can be given intravenously in a dose of 25–50 μg/kg but this is rarely necessary.

Atenolol
The main advantage of atenolol is that it can be given once a day, usually in a dose of 1 mg/kg. Tablets contain 25, 50, or 100 mg. A sugar-free syrup is available, containing 25 mg/5mL.

Nadolol
Nadolol is less often used but is the drug of choice for congenital long QT syndrome and catecholaminergic polymorphic ventricular tachycardia. It has a very long half-life and can be given once daily in a dose of 1 mg/kg. The 80-mg tablets can be halved and a liquid formulation is available for smaller children.

Sotalol
Sotalol differs from other β-blockers in that it is non-cardioselective and has additional class III (amiodarone-like) antiarrhythmic activity. It is mainly used for relatively rare atrial or ventricular arrhythmias. The dose is usually 2 mg/kg per day in two doses, sometimes increasing to 4 mg/kg per day.

Esmolol
Esmolol is only used intravenously and has a very short duration of action. It is used for termination of tachycardias and sometimes for short-term suppression. It is initially given in a dose of 500 μg/kg over 1 minute followed, if necessary, by an infusion of 50 μg/kg per min. This can be increased to 200 μg/kg per min.

Digoxin

Digoxin has relatively little direct antiarrhythmic effect and produces most of its effects through manipulation of the autonomic nervous system. It slows the sinus rate and AV nodal conduction, and prolongs AV nodal refactoriness. The refractory periods of the atria, ventricles, and accessory pathways are shortened. Digoxin has been used extensively in the past but is used less now that safer and more effective drugs are available. There is little objective evidence that it has a useful antiarrhythmic effect but it is included here for completeness. In the days when it was more widely used digoxin was the drug most commonly associated with prescription errors in pediatrics, with sometimes fatal consequences.

Indications

Digoxin is still used by some practitioners for suppression of some types of supraventricular tachycardia, particularly in infancy, and its effect on AV nodal conduction has been used for control of ventricular rate in various types of atrial tachycardia (β-blockers are now probably more effective but this is a rare indication in children).

Dosing

Quoted digitalizing doses are 20 µg/kg for preterm neonates, 30 µg/kg for term neonates, 40–50 µg/kg for infants, and 30–40 µg/kg for children aged <2 years. These doses are given orally over 24 hours in three divided doses. Maintenance doses, in micrograms/kilogram per day, are 5 and 8–10 µg/kg for preterm and term neonates, respectively, 10–12 µg/kg in infancy, and 8–10 µg/kg in children. These doses are intended to produce plasma levels of 1.1–1.7 µg/L. It is said that slightly higher levels may be required for arrhythmia control and are usually well tolerated.

Adverse effects

Toxic effect are rare at plasma levels <2 µg/L but are more common in the presence of hypokalemia. They include various types of bradycardia, AV block, or tachycardia as well as neurological and gastrointestinal symptoms. Digoxin interacts with other drugs, particularly verapamil and amiodarone, and doses may need to be adjusted.

Flecainide

Flecainide is a sodium channel blocker effective against a wide variety of arrhythmias. It has a narrower toxic therapeutic ratio than most other commonly used antiarrhythmic drugs in children, and attention should be paid to correct dosing and monitoring of plasma concentrations.

Indications

Flecainide is mainly used for control of AV re-entry tachycardia, incessant tachycardias such as permanent junctional reciprocating tachycardia and atrial ectopic tachycardia, and some types of ventricular tachycardia. It is best avoided in atrial flutter and postoperative atrial tachycardia because, by slowing the tachycardia, it can allow an increase in AV conduction and produce a paradoxical increase in ventricular rate.

Dosing

The effective oral dose in infants is usually in the range 6–8 mg/kg per day, in three divided doses. In children the dose is more often 3–6 mg/kg per day and twice daily dosing is usually effective. The plasma concentration should be checked after a few days – the therapeutic range is 250–750 µg/ml. It is recommended that treatment should be started in hospital. Infants and children with AV re-entry tachycardia should have a repeat ECG recorded before discharge because treatment can occasionally produce slower but incessant AV re-entry. Other proarrhythmia is rare. During follow-up the ECG may show minor QRS widening but, if this is marked or there is PR prolongation, it may be a sign of a high plasma concentration.

Flecainide is occasionally used intravenously with very close monitoring of the ECG, blood pressure, etc. It may be used for termination or rate control of intractable arrhythmias if ventricular function is not seriously impaired. It is given slowly over a few minutes in a dose of up to 2 mg/kg, depending on the response. Flecainide should only be given intravenously by those experienced in its use.

Propafenone

Propafenone is similar to flecainide in its effects and side effects but it also has some β-blocker activity. It is more widely used in some European countries. The indications for its use are similar to those for flecainide.

Dosing

Oral propafenone is effective in suppression of a variety of arrhythmias, usually given in a dose of 10–15 mg/kg per day in two or three doses. Propafenone can be given intravenously in a dose of 1–2 mg/kg, titrated against the response.

Verapamil

Verapamil is a calcium channel blocker and its main antiarrhythmic effect is suppression of AV nodal conduction. It is an effective drug used intravenously for termination of tachycardia in children but is contraindicated in infancy because it may cause bradycardia or cardiac arrest.

Indications

Verapamil is mostly used for termination of sustained tachycardias in which the AV node is part of the circuit – mainly AV nodal re-entry or AV re-entry tachycardias. It is occasionally used orally for suppression of rare arrhythmias such as posterior fascicular ventricular tachycardia (see Chapter 21) or permanent junctional reciprocating tachycardia (see Chapter 14).

Dosing

The intravenous dose is 100–300 μg/kg given slowly over a few minutes and stopping when the desired effect is achieved. The oral dose is usually 40–80 mg three times daily.

Adverse effects

Verapamil is avoided if ventricular function is poor or in patients also taking a β-blocker and in infants.

Conclusions

Drug treatment is only part of the management of an infant or child with a tachycardia. It is obviously important for the pediatrician or cardiologist to be familiar with the drug's dose, effects, and side effects. Before choosing a drug it is also important to consider the following:

- Is drug treatment the best option?
- Which drug is best?
- What is the correct dose?
- Is intravenous or oral treatment better?
- How should the response to treatment be monitored?
- For how long should treatment be continued?

Despite recent advances in non-pharmacological treatment of tachycardias, drug treatment remains an important part of the therapeutic plan for many children. It seems unlikely that there will be significant developments of new antiarrhythmic drugs in the near future, so we have a responsibility to use those currently available effectively and safely.

Key references

Burri S, Hug MI, Bauersfeld U. Efficacy and safety of intravenous amiodarone for incessant tachycardias in infants. *Eur J Pediatr* 2003;**162**:880–4.

Dixon J, Foster K, Wyllie J, et al. Guidelines and adenosine dosing for supraventricular tachycardia. *Arch Dis Child* 2005;**90**:1190–1.

Etheridge SP, Craig JE, Compton SJ. Amiodarone is safe and highly effective therapy for supraventricular tachycardia in infants. *Am Heart J* 2001;**141**:105–10.

Fenrich AL Jr, Perry JC, Friedman RA. Flecainide and amiodarone: combined therapy for refractory tachyarrhythmias in infancy. *J Am Coll Cardiol* 1995;**25**:1195–8.

Ferguson JD, DiMarco JP. Contemporary management of paroxysmal supraventricular tachycardia. *Circulation* 2003;**107**:1096–9.

Janoušek J, Paul T. Safety of oral propafenone in the treatment of arrhythmias in infants and children (European Retrospective Multicenter Study). *Am J Cardiol* 1998;**81**:1121–4.

Läer S, Elshoff JP, Meibohm B, et al. Development of a safe and effective pediatric dosing regimen for sotalol based on population pharmacokinetics and pharmacodynamics in children with supraventricular tachycardia. *J Am Coll Cardiol* 2005;**46**:1322–30.

O'Sullivan JJ, Gardiner HM, Wren C. Digoxin or flecainide for prophylaxis of supraventricular tachycardia in infants? *J Am Coll Cardiol* 1995;**26**:991–4.

Pfammatter JP, Bauersfeld U. Safety issues in the treatment of paediatric supraventricular tachycardias. *Drug Safety* 1998;**18**:345–56.

Price JF, Kertesz NJ, Snyder CS, et al. Flecainide and sotalol: a new combination therapy for refractory supraventricular tachycardia in children <1 year of age. *J Am Coll Cardiol* 2002;**39**:517–20.

Saul JP, Ross B, Schaffer MS, et al. Pharmacokinetics and pharmacodynamics of sotalol in a pediatric population with supraventricular and ventricular tachyarrhythmia. *Clin Pharmacol Ther* 2001;**69**:145–57.

Saul JP, Scott WA, Brown S, et al. Intravenous amiodarone for incessant tachyarrhythmias in children: a randomized, double-blind, antiarrhythmic drug trial. *Circulation* 2005;**112**:3470–7.

Saul JP, LaPage MJ. Is it time to tell the emperor he has no clothes?: Intravenous amiodarone for supraventricular arrhythmias in children. *Circ Arrhythm Electrophysiol* 2010;**3**:115–17.

Wong KK, Potts JE, Etheridge SP, et al. Medications used to manage supraventricular tachycardia in the infant. A North American Survey. *Pediatr Cardiol* 2006;**27**:199–203.

Wren C. Adenosine in paediatric arrhythmias. *Paediatr Perinat Drug Ther* 2006;**7**:114–17.

38 Pacemakers and implantable defibrillators

Pacing in children and adults with congenital heart disease is a large and complex subject so there is room here for only a very brief introduction. The interested reader is referred to the key references at the end of this section or to more specialized texts.

Pacemakers have been used in children since the early 1960s. Pediatric pacing started with external devices for children with postoperative complete atrioventricular (AV) block and developed with fully implantable devices. We now use very small reliable and long-lasting systems and can realistically contemplate a normal lifetime of pacing from birth in some patients (Figure 38.1).

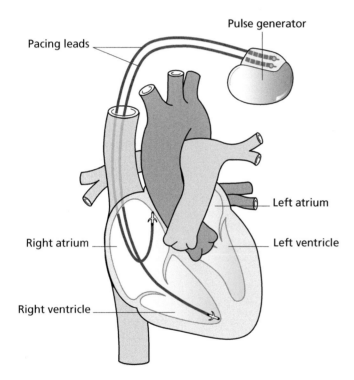

Figure 38.1

The basic concept of pacing is simple: pacemakers can do two things – sense and pace. Most work in demand mode; they will sense electrical activity in the atrium or ventricle and pace only if the next beat fails to arrive within a preset time period. The pacing output is usually in the range 1.5–4.5 V for 0.5–1.0 ms, which is usually adequate to capture the myocardium and produce a paced beat. Most pacemakers are rate responsive and can increase their rate in response to movement.

Concise Guide to Pediatric Arrhythmias, First Edition. Christopher Wren.
© 2012 John Wiley & Sons, Ltd. Published 2012 by John Wiley & Sons, Ltd.

Pacemaker leads

Pacemaker leads may be placed in the ventricle or atrium or both. Atrial pacing may be used to overcome bradycardia if AV conduction is known to be normal. Ventricular pacing is much more common and is used for treatment of AV block. It usually involves a VVIR pacing system (meaning that the generator paces the ventricle [V], senses the ventricle [V], is inhibited if it senses [I], and is rate responsive [R]). This system is simple and has only one lead (there is less to go wrong) but it does not provide AV synchrony. Dual-chamber pacing is routine in adult patients and in older children. It restores AV synchrony but involves insertion of two pacing leads. The most common would be a DDDR system, which paces or senses both chambers and can be either inhibited by or triggered by a sensed event and is rate responsive.

The two types of pacing lead employed are endocardial and epicardial. *Epicardial pacing* can be employed at any age and for more or less any complexity of cardiac malformation. Its disadvantages are that the leads are more prone to failure or fracture and the battery life is shorter. The radiograph in Figure 38.2 is from a neonate with an epicardial ventricular pacemaker.

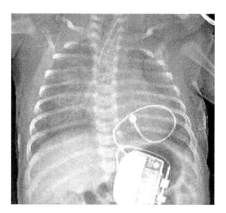

Figure 38.2

The advantage of *endocardial pacing* is that it is more reliable (lead failures are rare) and uses less energy, so generator life is prolonged. Its disadvantages are that it is more difficult to leave sufficient extra intravascular lead to allow for growth and the leads may cause venous occlusion, especially in infants and small children. It also presents practical difficulties in patients with a single ventricle circulation. Although endocardial pacing is feasible in the neonate, many units prefer epicardial pacing in small infants to be able to allow for growth and to reduce the risk of venous occlusion. The radiograph in Figure 38.3 is from a child with a dual chamber pacemaker. He has leads in the right atrium and right ventricle as well as the distal end of a previous epicardial lead. Figure 38.4 shows the radiograph of a 14-year-old boy who

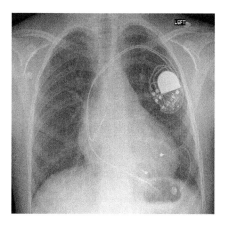

Figure 38.3

had a series of operations for complex transposition of the great arteries. In addition to right atrial and ventricular leads he has a third lead to pace the left ventricle via the coronary sinus to improve ventricular synchrony (red arrow). This produced a significant improvement in ventricular function.

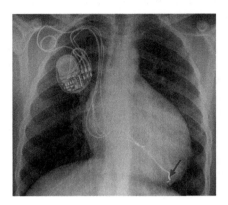

Figure 38.4

Pacing leads may be unipolar or bipolar, the latter being much more commonly used. Unipolar pacing systems are more susceptible to electrical interference from muscle movement. Bipolar leads are larger and produce a smaller pacing spike on the ECG. Most leads are steroid eluting, i.e. the tip contains a small pellet of dexamethasone that is released slowly and leads to a lower chronic pacing threshold.

Single-chamber pacing is the simplest system and is usually employed if the patient is small and there is good cardiac function. Dual-chamber pacing offers synchronized atrial and ventricular contraction. This is routinely employed in adults and older children, although the hemodynamic advantage over VVIR pacing in a patient with normal heart structure and function is small.

Pacemaker generators

The generator has a titanium casing and contains a lithium iodide battery. The battery life depends on several factors, including the pacing rate, voltage, and pulse width, and whether the system is pacing or sensing.

Indications for pacemaker implantation

The main indication for pacing in children is complete AV block (see Chapter 29), either congenital or acquired. Pacemaker implantation is also sometimes indicated for lesser degrees of block (see Chapter 28), for bradycardia in sinoatrial disease (see Chapter 30), or for resynchronization in heart failure.

The rhythm strip in Figure 38.5 shows VVI pacing via a single right ventricular lead. The ventricle is paced at a rate of 70/min and the sinus rhythm in the atrium remains dissociated.

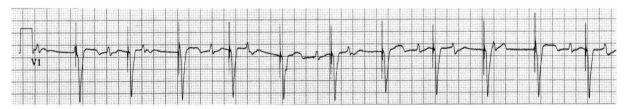

Figure 38.5

Figures 38.6 and 38.7 show DDD pacing. In each the P wave is sensed and the ventricle is paced after a preset AV delay, mimicking sinus rhythm.

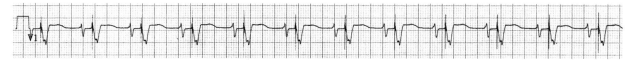

Figure 38.6

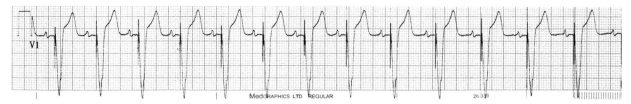

Figure 38.7

If the sinus rate is slower than the preset pacemaker rate the atrium and the ventricle will be paced with a preset AV delay, again mimicking sinus rhythm, as shown in Figure 38.8. The first pacing spike produces a P wave (black arrow), the second a QRS (red arrow).

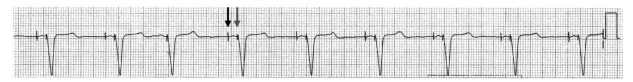

Figure 38.8

The ECG in Figure 38.9 shows a failure of the pacemaker system. The rhythm is sinus arrhythmia in the atria and there is a slow ventricular escape rhythm. Pacing spikes are seen but there is no capture (red arrows). This might be due to lead displacement or to exit block (a threshold higher than the pacemaker output) but in this case was due to a lead fracture.

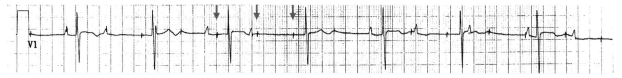

Figure 38.9

Outcome

Long-term reliable permanent pacing can be achieved in most infants and children. Early postoperative problems are uncommon but include infection, erosion, and exit block (a rise in threshold to higher than the pacemaker output). Lead survival is generally good and is better for endocardial leads. Children with pacemakers require follow-up every 6 months or so to measure the lead threshold, check the sensing, and estimate the remaining generator life. The characteristics of rate response can be adjusted for optimum performance.

Resynchronization

Cardiac resynchronization therapy (CRT) can be used as part of the treatment of heart failure associated with ventricular dyssynchrony in patients with pediatric or congenital heart disease. It involves pacing both ventricles to correct dyssynchrony of the systemic ventricle (usually the left). That entails pacing the left ventricle either via a lead in the coronary sinus or epicardially. At best CRT can return cardiac function to nearly normal and defer listing for heart transplantation. Resynchronization may be helpful in association with surgery for tricuspid regurgitation in some patients with a failing systemic right ventricle.

Implantable defibrillators

In recent years implantable cardioverter–defibrillators (ICDs) have been used widely in adult patients but their use in children is very limited. This is mainly because life-threatening arrhythmias unsuitable for other forms of antiarrhythmic treatment are rare in children and because of the significant technical difficulties of ICD implantation in small children. An ICD is similar to a large pacemaker and is implanted in patients at risk of sudden death from ventricular fibrillation or ventricular tachycardia. It is designed to sense these two arrhythmias and to deliver a DC shock, usually of 17–40 J, to restore sinus rhythm. ICD implantation in children presents more challenges than pacemaker implantation because the devices are larger and the leads longer and less adaptable to small or malformed hearts. Epicardial systems are now rarely used and subcutaneous systems may offer some promise in the future.

The main indications for ICD implantation are refractory ventricular arrhythmias in conditions such as congenital long QT syndrome, catecholaminergic polymorphic ventricular tachycardia, and Brugada syndrome. They are also used in adults with repaired congenital heart disease and a high risk of sudden death. They are of proven benefit in secondary prevention in hypertrophic cardiomyopathy but their role in primary prevention has been difficult to define.

Compared with adult practice, ICD implantation in children and adults with congenital heart disease is associated with a higher rate of complications such as infections, lead dislodgement, and lead failure from either insulation breaches or conductor breaks. It also presents greater difficulties with device programming and there is a higher rate of inappropriate shocks.

ICD implantation imposes a significant psychological burden on the child and family. Inappropriate shocks are frightening and lead malfunctions can be demoralizing, especially if the ICD was implanted for primary prevention and has not been needed for an appropriate shock.

ICD lead selection depends on the patient's clinical profile. With a single-coil lead the current travels from the coil to the device metal can. With a dual-coil lead the shock follows two pathways: from the ventricular (distal) coil to the proximal coil, and from the distal coil to the device can. Dual-coil leads have slightly lower defibrillation thresholds but extraction of a dual-coil lead is likely to be more difficult.

The radiograph in Figure 38.10 shows an ICD in a 15-year-old girl with Brugada syndrome. She has a single-coil lead and a subpectoral generator.

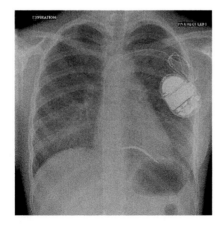

Figure 38.10

The X-ray in Figure 38.11 shows an ICD in a 13-year-old boy with severe hypertrophic cardiomyopathy. He has a dual-coil lead and an atrial pacing lead to provide dual chamber pacing. The generator is subpectoral.

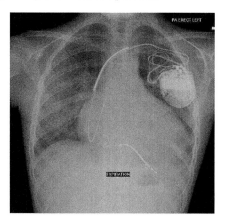

Figure 38.11

The radiograph in Figure 38.12 shows an ICD in a 16 kg boy with congenital long QT syndrome and recurrent torsades de pointes despite high dose β-blocker treatment. ICD implantation in children of this size presents considerable technical difficulties. He has a unipolar system with a single coil in the right ventricle. The lead was introduced via the left subclavian vein and tunneled subcutaneously to the generator in a pocket behind rectus abdominis in the anterior abdominal wall. The recording in Figure 38.13, from the same boy, shows an appropriate DC shock terminating a prolonged episode of torsades de pointes. The device has detected the arrhythmia and delivered a shock of 17 J. Temporary ventricular pacing takes over after 2 s because of post-shock bradycardia.

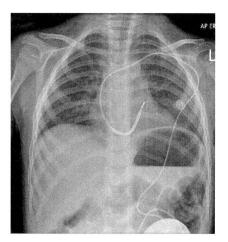

Figure 38.12

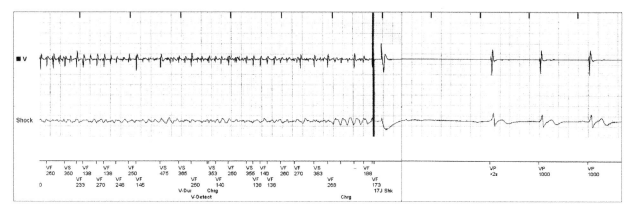

Figure 38.13

Key references

Berul CI. Implantable cardioverter defibrillator criteria for primary and secondary prevention of pediatric sudden cardiac death. *Pacing Clin Electrophysiol* 2008;**32**(suppl 2):S67–70.

Berul CI, Van Hare GF, Kertesz NJ, et al. Results of a multicenter retrospective implantable cardioverter–defibrillator registry of pediatric and congenital heart disease patients. *J Am Coll Cardiol* 2008;**51**:1685–91.

Blom NA. Implantable cardioverter–defibrillators in children. *Pacing Clin Electrophysiol* 2008;**31**(suppl 1):S32–4.

Cecchin F, Atallah J, Walsh EP, Triedman JK, Alexander ME, Berul CI. Lead extraction in pediatric and congenital heart disease patients/clinical perspective. *Circ Arrhythm Electrophysiol* 2010;**3**:5437–44.

Epstein AE, DiMarco JP, Ellenbogen KA, et al. ACC/AHA/HRS 2008 Guidelines for device-based therapy of cardiac rhythm abnormalities: a report of the American College of Cardiology/American Heart Association Task Force on Practice Guidelines. *Circulation* 2008;**117**:e350–408.

Janousek J, Gebauer RA, Abdul-Khaliq H, et al. Cardiac resynchronisation therapy in paediatric and congenital heart disease: differential effects in various anatomical and functional substrates. *Heart* 2009;**95**:1165–71.

Janousek J. Cardiac resynchronisation in congenital heart disease. *Heart* 2009;**95**:940–7.

Karpawich PP. Technical aspects of pacing in adult and pediatric congenital heart disease. *Pacing Clin Electrophysiol* 2008;**31**(suppl 1):S28–31.

McLeod KA. Cardiac pacing in infants and children. *Heart* 2010;**96**:1502–8.

Rajappan K. Permanent pacemaker implantation technique: part I. *Heart* 2009;**95**;259–64.

Rajappan K. Permanent pacemaker implantation technique: part II. *Heart* 2009;**95**;334–42.

Roberts PR. Follow up and optimisation of cardiac pacing. *Heart* 2005;**91**:1229–34.

Schwartz PJ, Spazzolini C, Priori SG, et al. Who are the long-QT syndrome patients who receive an implantable cardioverter–defibrillator and what happens to them? *Circulation* 2010;**122**:1272–82.

Vardas PE, Auricchio A, Blanc JJ, et al. Guidelines for cardiac pacing and cardiac resynchronization therapy: the task force for cardiac pacing and cardiac resynchronization therapy of the European Society of Cardiology. *Eur Heart J* 2007;**28**:2256–95.

Villain E. Indications for pacing in patients with congenital heart disease. *Pacing Clin Electrophysiol* 2008;**31**(suppl 1):S17–20.

Walsh EP. Practical aspects of implantable defibrillator therapy in patients with congenital heart disease. *Pacing Clin Electrophysiol* 2008;**31**(suppl 1):S38–40.

Wilkoff BL, Love CJ, Byrd CL, et al. Transvenous lead extraction: Heart Rhythm Society expert consensus on facilities, training, indications, and patient management. *Heart Rhythm* 2009;**6**:1085–104.

39 Catheter ablation

The options for management of tachycardia were changed dramatically about 20 years ago by the introduction of catheter ablation. Until then antiarrhythmic drugs had been the mainstay of treatment, with a direct surgical approach reserved for the most intractable arrhythmias. Now most common tachycardias are amenable to radiofrequency ablation, so many children have a realistic prospect of a non-surgical cure. In experienced hands the procedure has a high success rate and low complication rate, and is preferred to long-term antiarrhythmic drug treatment or continuing symptoms. It is used less often in infants and small children mainly because of the high rate of spontaneous resolution of their arrhythmias, partly because of the technical difficulty of adapting the technique to small children and also because of some concern about the possible long-term sequelae of ablation lesions in those with very small hearts.

Radiofrequency catheter ablation involves delivery of an electric current to a focal point of myocardium at around 500 kHz, usually using a temperature of around 60°C, and delivering energy of 50–100 W. The ablation produces a lesion a few millimeters wide and deep. If this is accurately positioned it can destroy the substrate for the arrhythmia (Figure 39.1). If the target for ablation is in an unusual position, such as an accessory pathway in the coronary sinus or one of its branches, energy delivery may be too low using conventional temperature-limited ablation. This is overcome by using an irrigated catheter to limit the catheter tip temperature rise and allow greater energy delivery. The lesion produced is governed by the energy delivered (to induce a rise in tissue temperature immediately adjacent to the catheter tip) rather than by the catheter tip temperature itself.

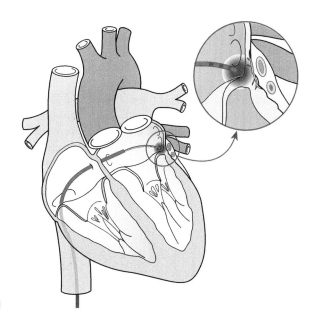

Figure 39.1

Concise Guide to Pediatric Arrhythmias, First Edition. Christopher Wren.
© 2012 John Wiley & Sons, Ltd. Published 2012 by John Wiley & Sons, Ltd.

Success rates and complications

The immediate success rate for catheter ablation of tachycardia mediated by a left-sided accessory pathway exceeds 95%, and the recurrence rate in the few months after the procedure should be no more than 5%. Late recurrence is rare. Most operators prefer a transseptal approach to left-sided pathways if there is no foramen ovale and use of the retrograde transaortic approach is unusual. The success rate for right-sided pathways is a little lower, partly because a few are very close to the bundle of His or atrioventricular (AV) node and partly because access to right-sided pathways is occasionally difficult. The main concern over accessory pathway ablation is the risk of producing AV block but the risk is low. Cryoablation is said to be a safer procedure for pathways close to the normal conduction axis but has a higher recurrence rate. Other complications are uncommon. Minor complications include vascular trauma, hematoma, and bleeding. Major complications, such as cardiac perforation, valve trauma, damage to the coronary arteries, and systemic embolism, are rare.

Figure 39.2 shows the ECG during ablation of a right-sided accessory pathway in a 5-year-old child with Wolff–Parkinson–White syndrome. Ablation is performed in sinus rhythm so that the disappearance of the delta wave can be observed. In Figure 39.2 the first six beats show a large delta wave and the last four are normal.

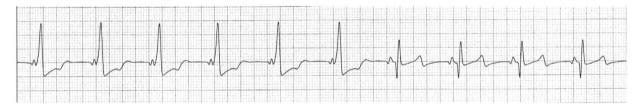

Figure 39.2

Ablation of the more common concealed accessory pathway is usually performed during right ventricular pacing, so that the block in retrograde ventriculoatrial conduction can be observed.

In children with AV nodal re-entrant tachycardia, the target for ablation is the "slow pathway" in the posteroseptal region of the tricuspid annulus. After preliminary electrophysiology study, ablation is performed in sinus rhythm, and repeat electrophysiology study is required to test the efficacy. The aim is to modify AV node function without producing AV block. Experience has shown that this can usually be achieved and the expected success rate should exceed 90%. The major complication is production of complete AV block requiring pacemaker implantation (with a quoted risk of up to 1%). The recurrence rate depends on the operator but is usually 5–10%. Again cryoablation may be safer but has a significant recurrence rate.

The reported success of ablation of focal atrial tachycardia varies, depending partly on the site of the tachycardia, but is generally in the range 80–90%. Recurrence after acute success is unusual. Figure 39.3 shows the ECG during ablation of left atrial tachycardia in a 10-year-old boy with severely impaired ventricular function. As the arrhythmia is incessant, ablation is performed in tachycardia. The change in P wave morphology from tachycardia (black arrow) to sinus rhythm (red arrow) is more obvious in lead aVF than V1. The ventricular function returned to normal within 3 months.

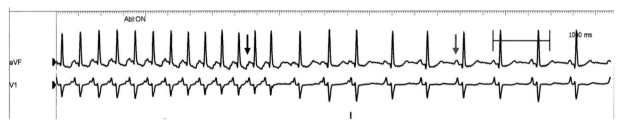

Figure 39.3

Catheter ablation of other atrial arrhythmias, such as atrial flutter, is mostly confined to late postoperative arrhythmias. The success rate depends mainly on the substrate but also on the experience and perseverance of the operator. Good results are reported for ablation of atrial flutter late after repair of a tetralogy of Fallot and in expert hands these can nearly be matched in patients with a Senning or Mustard repair of transposition of the great arteries. Ablation of atrial arrhythmias in patients with a Fontan palliation of single ventricle is a more disappointing and frustrating procedure, mainly because of the substrate – the right atrium may be hugely dilated and the atrial wall is hypertrophied and scarred with adherent mural thrombus. Ablation of this type of tachycardia cannot be achieved with one or two focal lesions and is done by producing long linear lesions to destroy re-entry circuits.

Other arrhythmias are also amenable to catheter ablation but the numbers reported are small, and it can be difficult to get a true picture of the success rate. Having said that, success is common and serious complications are rare. These arrhythmias include atriofascicular re-entry (with an unusual accessory connection on the lateral aspect of the tricuspid valve – see Chapter 15), permanent junctional re-entry tachycardia (with a slowly conducting concealed accessory pathway close to the mouth of the coronary sinus – see Chapter 14), left posterior fascicular ventricular tachycardia (see Chapter 21), and right ventricular outflow tachycardia (see Chapter 22). Figure 39.4 shows ablation of permanent junctional reciprocating tachycardia in a 4-year-old girl. Tachycardia stops within 3 s of the start of energy delivery but ablation is continued for 60 s to ensure a permanent effect. The change in P wave morphology from tachycardia (black arrow) to sinus rhythm (red arrow) as tachycardia stops is obvious.

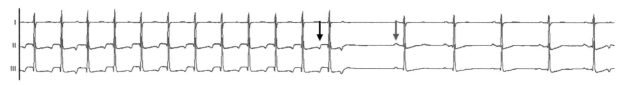

Figure 39.4

Key references

Aliot EM, Stevenson WG, Almendral-Garrote JM, et al. EHRA/HRS expert consensus on catheter ablation of ventricular arrhythmias. *Europace* 2009;**11**:771–817.

LaPage MJ, Saul JP, Reed JH. Long-term outcomes for cryoablation of pediatric patients with atrioventricular nodal reentrant tachycardia. *Am J Cardiol* 2010;**105**:1118–21.

Triedman J, Perry J, Van Hare G. Risk stratification for prophylactic ablation in asymptomatic Wolff–Parkinson–White syndrome. *N Engl J Med* 2005;**352**:92–3.

Van Hare GF, Colan SD, Javitz H, et al. Prospective assessment after pediatric cardiac ablation: fate of intracardiac structure and function, as assessed by serial echocardiography. *Am Heart J* 2007;**153**:815–20.

Van Hare GF. Pediatric electrophysiology series – catheter ablation in children. Heart Rhythm 2009;**6**:423–5.

Walsh EP. Interventional electrophysiology in patients with congenital heart disease. *Circulation* 2007;**115**:3224–34.

40 Artifacts

ECG artifacts can simulate a variety of cardiac arrhythmias, usually atrial or ventricular tachycardia. Artifacts may be seen on 12-lead or ambulatory ECGs. They are most often due to poor skin–electrode contact or interference from movement or tremor. Figure 40.1 shows an ECG from a 13-year-old girl who had had repair of a tetralogy of Fallot in infancy. The QRS complexes are irregular and in most leads the rhythm looks like atrial fibrillation. However, in lead II, and in the chest leads, she is clearly in sinus rhythm with respiratory sinus arrhythmia.

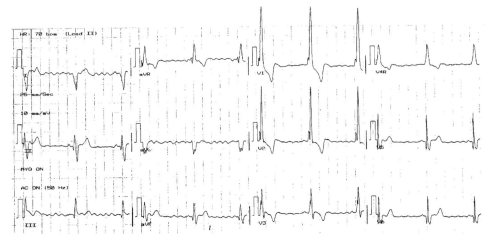

Figure 40.1

Figure 40.2 shows another movement artifact in an infant being patted by its mother for comfort during the recording. This looks almost like polymorphic ventricular tachycardia in some leads. Notice that lead III and most of the chest leads are not affected. This presumably means that the mechanical stimulation mostly affected the right arm lead.

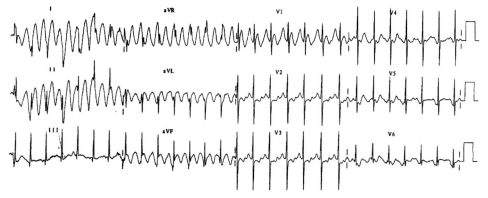

Figure 40.2

Figure 40.3 is a Holter recording of an infant with complete atrioventricular block. The apparent wide QRS tachycardia is again an artifact caused by the infant being patted by the mother.

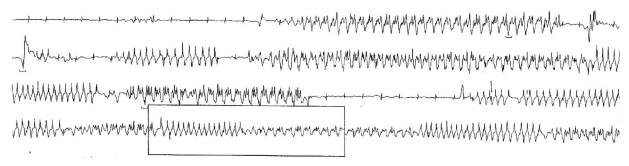

Figure 40.3

The ECG in Figure 40.4 is from a child with hiccoughs. The rhythm strip from lead V1 at first glance shows regular ventricular premature beats. However, on closer inspection these "beats" have a very strange morphology, do not disturb sinus rhythm, have QRS complexes superimposed on them (red arrows), and, most importantly, are really seen only in lead V1. Presumably the lead V1 electrode or its connection was loose to make it affected by the movement.

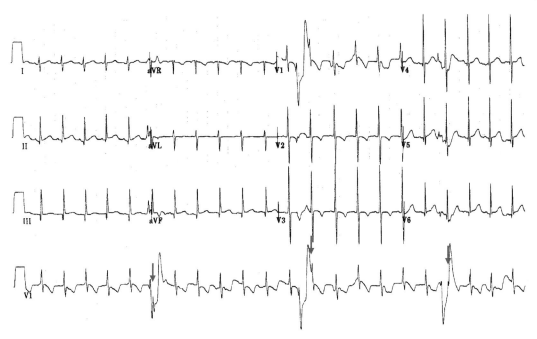

Figure 40.4

Figure 40.5 shows another movement artifact, this time mimicking ventricular tachycardia in an infant with a tetralogy of Fallot who was being patted by the mother. Note that the QRS complexes "walk through" the apparent ventricular tachycardia (arrows).

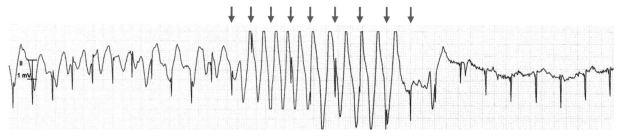

Figure 40.5

The intriguing appearance in Figure 40.6 is not really an artifact but may be seen after orthotopic heart transplantation. There are two sets of P waves, some of which are clearly related to the QRS complexes (black arrows), so this is obviously sinus rhythm and they come from the donor atrium. The other P waves (red arrows) have a different shape and are dissociated from sinus rhythm – they come from the original recipient atrium.

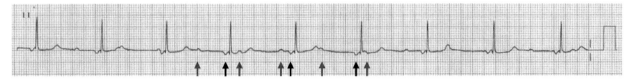

Figure 40.6

The ECG in Figure 40.7 comes from a boy who received a heterotopic ("piggy-back") heart transplant. There are two superimposed sets of QRS complexes. The smaller deflections are from the native heart and the larger complexes from the donor heart.

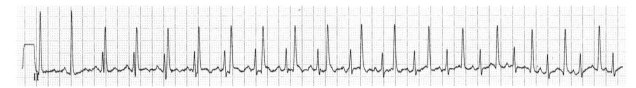

Figure 40.7

Key references

Brouillette RT, Thach BT, Abu-Osba YK, et al. Hiccups in infants: characteristics and effects on ventilation. *J Pediatr* 1980;**96**:219–25.

Knight BP, Pelosi F, Michaud GF, et al. Clinical consequences of electrocardiographic artifact mimicking ventricular tachycardia. *N Engl J Med* 1999;**341**:1270–4.

Srikureja W, Darbar D, Reeder GS. Tremor-induced artifact mimicking ventricular tachycardia. *Circulation* 2000;**102**:1337–8.

Tarkin JM, Hadjiloizou N, Kaddoura S, et al. Variable presentation of ventricular tachycardia-like electrocardiographic artifacts. *J Electrocardiol* 2010;**43**:691–3.

Appendix

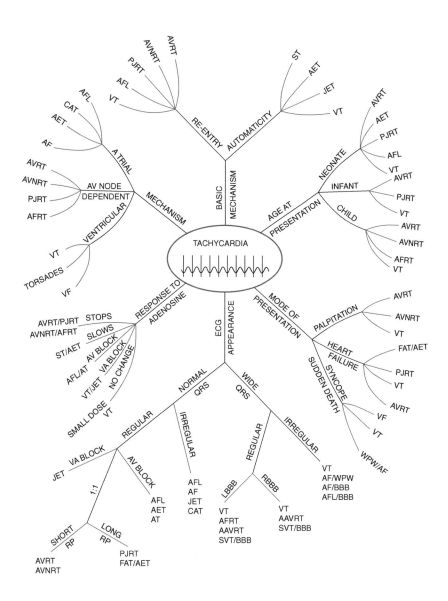

Concise Guide to Pediatric Arrhythmias, First Edition. Christopher Wren.
© 2012 John Wiley & Sons, Ltd. Published 2012 by John Wiley & Sons, Ltd.

Index

Note: Page numbers with italicized *f*'s and *t*'s refer to figures and tables, respectively.

Concise Guide to Pediatric Arrhythmias, First Edition. Christopher Wren.
© 2012 John Wiley & Sons, Ltd. Published 2012 by John Wiley & Sons, Ltd.

Printed and bound by CPI Group (UK) Ltd, Croydon, CR0 4YY

09/01/2024

08219934-0001
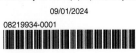